CHILDHOOD OBESITY

LICENSE, DISCLAIMER OF LIABILITY, AND LIMITED WARRANTY

CHILDHOOD OBESITY

Rita Buckley

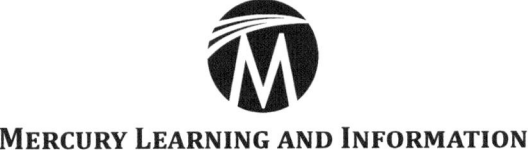

MERCURY LEARNING AND INFORMATION

Dulles, Virginia
Boston, Massachusetts
New Delhi

Portions of this book originally appeared or have been adapted from:

Heart Disease and Health. Dr. G. Gadkari and J. Larsen. ©2014 by Mercury Learning and Information. All rights reserved.

Obesity. Dr. G. Gadkari and E. Coveney. ©2014 by Mercury Learning and Information. All rights reserved.

Publisher: David Pallai
MERCURY LEARNING AND INFORMATION
22841 QUICKSILVER DRIVE
Dulles, VA 20166
info@merclearning.com
www.merclearning.com
(800) 232-0223

This book is printed on acid-free paper.

Rita Buckley. *Childhood Obesity.*
ISBN: 978-1-937585-42-6

Library of Congress Control Number: 2014950124
1516 17 3 2 1   Printed in the United States of America

Our titles are available for adoption, license, or bulk purchase by institutions, corporations, etc. For additional information, please contact the Customer Service Dept. at (800)232-0223(toll free).

All of our titles are available in digital format at authorcloudware.com and other digital vendors. Companion disc files for this title are available by contacting info@merclearning.com. The sole obligation of MERCURY LEARNING AND INFORMATION to the purchaser is to replace the disc, based on defective materials or faulty workmanship, but not based on the operation or functionality of the product.

Contents

PART ONE — **Childhood Obesity Basics**

CHAPTER 1 — *Childhood Obesity and Its Causes*

CHAPTER 2 — *Childhood Obesity and Health*

CHAPTER 3 — *Assessing Risk for Obesity in Children*

CHAPTER 4

Preventing Childhood Obesity

Preventing Obesity in Infants (0 to 12 Months)

Preventing Obesity in Toddlers (12 to 36 Months)

CHAPTER 8   *Preventing Obesity in Adolescence*

Assessing and Treating Obesity

The Role of the Physician in Childhood Obesity

Acknowledgments

My thanks to my publisher, David Pallai, my dear friend and mentor, George L. Blackburn, M.D., Ph.D., and my mother, Vera Swartz.

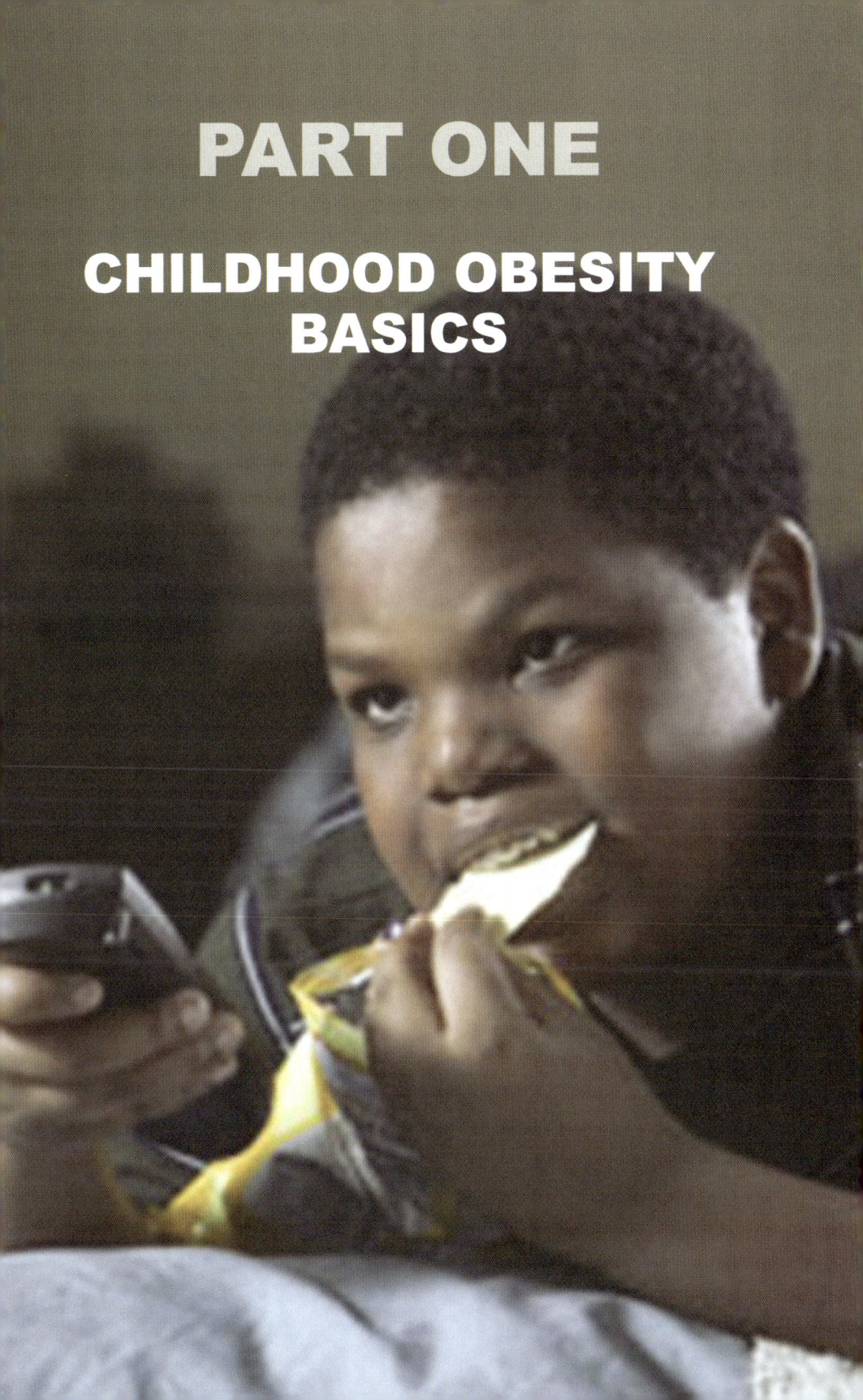

PART ONE

CHILDHOOD OBESITY BASICS

In Part One, we define childhood obesity and show you how it's measured in infants and toddlers as well as children and adolescents. We cover growth charts and how to calculate your child's body mass index (BMI), the measure used to determine obesity in youth 2–19 years of age. We then talk about the main causes of childhood obesity, its prevalence, and economic costs. A discussion of childhood obesity and health follows, including why obesity is a public health problem and its physical, psychological, and academic effects. Finally, we examine how to assess risk for childhood obesity.

CHAPTER 1
Childhood Obesity and Its Causes

CHAPTER 2
Childhood Obesity and Health

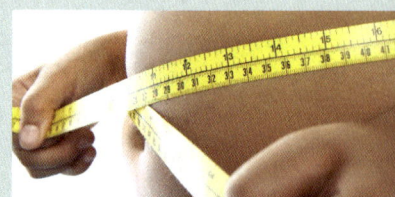

CHAPTER 3
Assessing Risk for Obesity in Children

Childhood Obesity and Its Causes

1. What is childhood obesity?

Childhood obesity is a worldwide epidemic. In the United States alone, approximately 17% (or 12.5 million) of children and adolescents aged 2–19 years are obese. Globally, the situation is equally dire, with prevalence increasing at an alarming rate.

In 2010, the number of overweight children under the age of five was estimated to be over 42 million.[1] To cope with the great numbers of affected youth, emphasis on obesity prevention during early childhood has become a priority; one that has finally paid off

Obesity is defined as abnormal or excessive fat accumulation that presents a risk to health.

with substantial success in children aged 2–5 years, a small but important slice of the American population. In this group, the obesity rate has dropped 43% over the past decade.[2]

Childhood obesity has been associated with cardiovascular disease risk factors, increased health-care costs, and premature death. The high toll it exacts from individuals and nations makes it one of the greatest public health challenges of the twenty-first century.

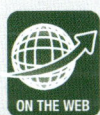

For an overview of what has caused the childhood obesity crisis and what we need to do to fight it, see Video 1.1: What Is It?

2. What is the prevalence of childhood obesity?

In the United States, recent years have seen little or no change in the prevalence of childhood obesity, and rates remain very high. The latest figures show that 8.1% of infants and toddlers were obese in 2011–2012 and 7.1% were severely obese. During the same period of time, 17% of children aged 2–19 years were obese.[3] Severe or extreme obesity is the fastest growing subcategory of obesity in children and adolescents.

3. What are the main causes of childhood obesity?

The main cause of childhood obesity is energy imbalance: eating too many calories and not getting enough physical activity.

Many factors fuel this imbalance, such as a lack of physical education in schools, not getting 60 minutes of physical activity a day, and overweight teens who consume 700 to 1,000 more calories per day than what they need to be healthy and fit. Over the course of 10 years, this excess can pack on 57 unnecessary pounds.[4]

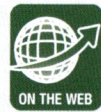

In America, youth aged 8–18 years spend 7.5 hours a day watching TV or playing video or computer games—3.5 times the limit recommended by the Academy of Pediatrics.

4. What is the annual economic toll from childhood obesity?

Childhood obesity alone is responsible for $14 billion in direct annual medical costs. Overall, these expenses are likely to rise significantly, especially if today's obese children become tomorrow's obese adults.

5. What are growth charts and how are they used?

Growth charts are a series of percentile curves that show the distribution of selected body measurements in U.S. children between 2–19 years of age. From birth up to 23 months, obesity is determined by length-for-age and weight-for-age percentiles. Updated guidelines from the Centers for Disease Control and Prevention (CDC) call for use of the World Health Organization (WHO) growth charts for children up to 23 months of age and the CDC growth charts for children 2 years and older.

To see a WHO growth chart for boys up to 23 months of age, visit:

www.cdc.gov/growthcharts/data/who/grchrt_boys_24lw_100611.pdf

To see a WHO growth chart for girls up to 23 months of age, visit:

http://www.cdc.gov/growthcharts/data/who/grchrt_girls_24lw_9210.pdf

The 2000 CDC growth charts consist of a total of 16 charts (8 for boys and 8 for girls), including two BMI-for-age charts for children and adolescents aged 2–20 years.

BMI-for-age charts are a major new addition to the CDC pediatric growth charts. They can be used to calculate and plot body mass index (BMI). However, they are not meant to be used as a diagnostic method. Rather, BMI-for-age charts are tools that contribute to an overall clinical impression of a child.

6. How do the WHO growth charts work?

The WHO charts reflect growth patterns among children mainly breastfed for at least four months and still breastfeeding at twelve months. They describe the growth of healthy children living in well-supported environments in six countries, including the United States. The charts show how infants and children should grow rather than simply how they do so in a certain time and place, and their use is therefore recommended for all infants.[5]

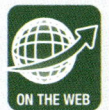

For BMI-for-age charts for boys 2–20 years of age, visit:

http://www.cdc.gov/growthcharts/data/set1clinical/cj41cs023c.pdf

For BMI-for-age charts for girls 2–20 years of age, visit:

http://www.cdc.gov/growthcharts/data/set1clinical/cj41cs024c.pdf

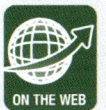

To watch a girl grow up in two minutes, see Video 1.2: Two-Minute Growth.

The charts also establish the growth of the breastfed infant as the norm. Healthy breastfed infants typically put on weight more slowly than formula-fed infants in the first year of life. Infants fed formula gain weight more rapidly after around three months of age. Differences in weight patterns continue even after complementary foods are introduced.

7. What is BMI?

Body mass index is a number calculated from a child's weight and height. It is defined as body weight in kilograms divided by height in meters squared:

$$BMI = weight\ (kg)/height\ (m)^2$$

BMI is the commonly accepted index for classifying adiposity or fatness in adults; it is also recommended for use with children and adolescents. It is consistent with adult BMI, and can be used to track body size throughout the life cycle. Like growth charts, BMI is not a diagnostic tool but is used to screen individuals who are underweight or overweight.

BMI is an indirect measure of body fat rather than a direct one, such as dual energy x-ray absorptiometry, which is a technique that is mostly used in research studies to confirm the accuracy of other ways to measure body fat. BMI is a reliable indicator for most children and teens and can be used as a proxy for direct measures. It is also an inexpensive and easy way to screen for weight categories that might lead to health problems. Fatness varies with age and sex during childhood and adolescence. Accordingly, BMI is age- and sex-specific. It is often referred to as BMI-for-age.

8. Can I find out if my child or teen is obese by using an adult BMI calculator?

The answer is no. The adult calculator only provides the BMI number, not the age- and sex-specific percentiles that are used to interpret BMI and determine the weight category for children and teens. It is inappropriate to use BMI categories for adults to interpret BMI numbers for children or adolescents. However, the CDC has developed a BMI Percentile Calculator for children and teens. If your child's height and weight are accurately measured, it will give you a BMI and the corresponding BMI-for-age percentile on a CDC BMI-for-age growth chart.

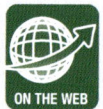

For information on how to accurately measure your child's height and weight at home, visit:

http://www.cdc.gov/healthyweight/assessing/bmi/childrens_BMI/measuring_children.html

For the child and teen BMI Percentile Calculator, visit:

http://apps.nccd.cdc.gov/dnpabmi/

The child and teen BMI Percentile Calculator should only be used for youth aged 2-19 years.

9. What is a BMI percentile?

BMI percentiles are the most commonly used clinical indicator to assess the size and growth patterns of children in the United States. Percentiles rank a child by indicating what percent of the reference population he or she equals or exceeds. After a clinician calculates a BMI for a child or teen, the BMI number is plotted on the CDC BMI-for-age growth charts (for either girls or boys) to obtain a percentile ranking. The percentile indicates the relative position of the child's BMI number among youngsters of the same sex and age. For example, on the weight-for-age growth charts, a 5-year-old girl whose weight is at the 25th percentile weighs the same or more than 25% of the reference population of 5-year-old girls and less than 75% of the 5-year-old girls (see Section 8).

Using the BMI Percentile Calculator involves the following steps:

1. Before calculating BMI, obtain accurate height and weight measurements of your child or teen (see Section 8).

2. Calculate the BMI and percentile using the child and teen BMI Percentile Calculator (see Section 8). The BMI number is calculated using standard formulas.

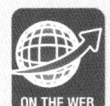

To see the standard formulas, visit:

ON THE WEB   http://www.cdc.gov/
healthyweight/
assessing/bmi/childrens_bmi/
childrens_bmi_formula.html

3. Review the calculated BMI-for-age percentile and results. The BMI-for-age percentile is used to interpret the BMI number, which is both age- and sex-specific for children and teens. Age and sex are considered for children and teens for two reasons:

   • The amount of body fat changes with age.
   • The amount of body fat differs between girls and boys.

The CDC BMI-for-age growth charts for boys and girls take these differences into account and allow translation of a BMI number into a percentile based on the sex and age of a child or teen (see Section 5 and 9).

4. Find the weight status category for the calculated BMI-for-age percentile as shown in the following table. These categories are based on expert committee recommendations.

BMI-for-age weight categories and percentile ranges.

WEIGHT STATUS CATEGORY	PERCENTILE RANGE
Underweight	Less than the 5th percentile
Healthy weight	5th percentile to less than the 85th percentile
Overweight	85th to less than the 95th percentile
Obese	Equal to or greater than the 95th percentile

SOURCE: CDC, About BMI for Children and Teens

http://www.cdc.gov/healthyweight/assessing/bmi/childrens_bmi/about_childrens_bmi.html

The following example shows a BMI-for-age analysis for a 10-year-old boy.

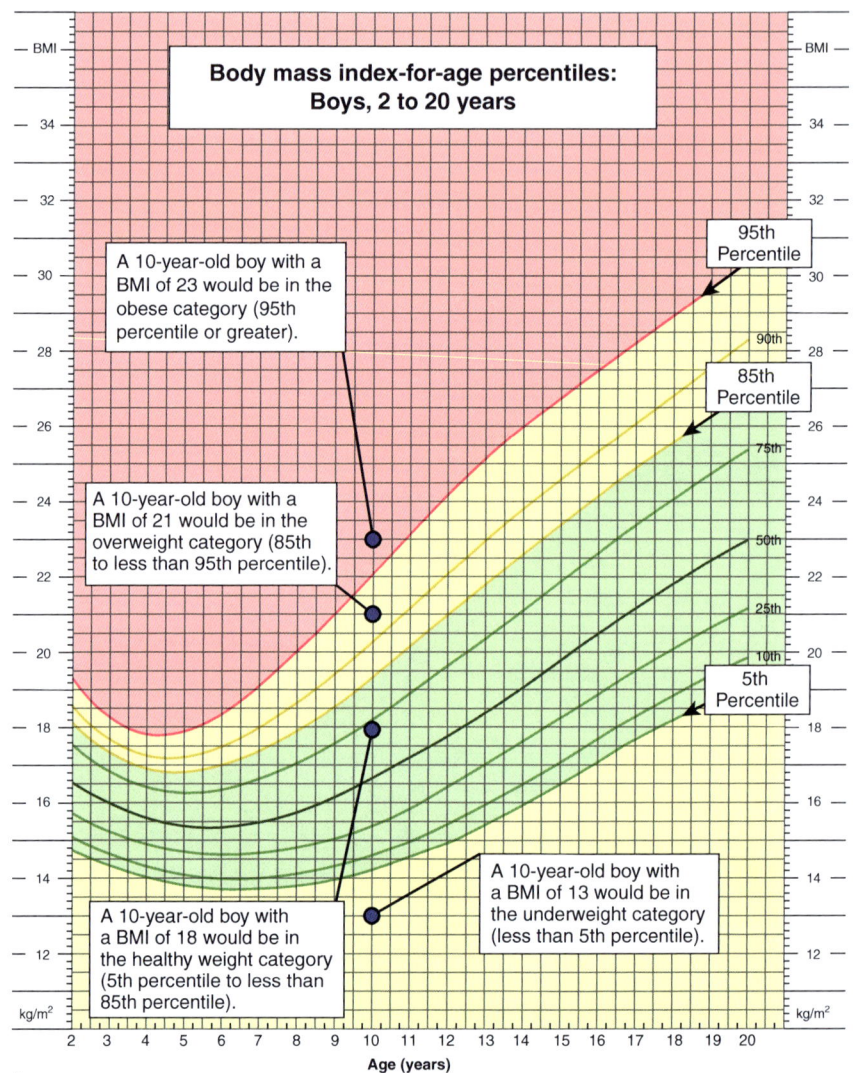

FIGURE 1.1
Percentile rank indicates body mass index (BMI) equal to or exceeded by the age of the reference population.

11. How can I tell if my child is obese?

The CDC and the American Academy of Pediatrics recommend the use of BMI to screen for obesity in children and teens aged 2–19 years. BMI is not a diagnostic tool. For example, a child who is relatively heavy may have a high BMI for his or her age. To determine if the child has excess fat, further assessment might include skinfold thickness measurements, magnetic resonance imaging (MRI), or computed tomography (CT) scanning.

Children less than 2 years of age are at risk for overweight if their growth measurements are between the 84.1st and 97.7th percentiles of the WHO growth charts (see Section 6).

12. What is adiposity rebound?

BMI changes substantially with age. After about one year of age, BMI-for-age begins to decline. It continues to fall during the preschool years until it reaches a minimum at around four to six years of age. After that time, it begins a gradual increase through adolescence and most of adulthood. The rebound or increase in BMI that occurs after it reaches its lowest point is referred to as adiposity rebound. This is a normal pattern of growth that occurs in all children.

Childhood obesity is a BMI at or above the 95th percentile for children of the same age and sex. For example, a 3-year-old boy of average height who weighs more than 37 pounds would be considered obese.

Extreme or severe obesity is defined as a BMI at or above 120% of the 95th percentile for children of the same age and sex. For example, a 3-year-old boy of average height who weighs more than 44 pounds would be classified as extremely obese.

Adiposity rebound is a period of increasing BMI after the early childhood low point, usually at about six years old.

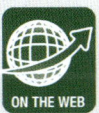

For a short talk on the meaning of adiposity or BMI rebound, visit:

http://www.healthychildren.org/English/health-issues/conditions/obesity/pages/BMI-Rebound-An-Obesity-Clue.aspx

Childhood Obesity and Health

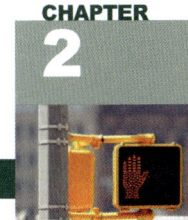

CHAPTER 2

13. Is childhood obesity a disease?

The American Medical Association (AMA) officially recognized obesity as a disease in 2013. The group's decision is likely to focus more attention on obesity and prompt physicians to take steps to screen, prevent, and treat it. It will also put pressure on health insurance companies to pay for obesity drugs, surgery, and counseling. Perhaps it will help reduce the shame and stigma that comes from a widespread notion that being obese is a lifestyle decision, just a matter of eating too much and not exercising enough. A large body of scientific and clinical evidence shows otherwise: individuals do not have full control over their weight.

To see the AMA resolution, visit:

http://media.npr.org/documents/2013/jun/ama-resolution-obesity.pdf

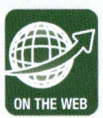

14. Why can't kids just outgrow it?

Excess weight-for-length isn't just baby fat, something infants and toddlers will outgrow over time. The first years of life are critically important to a child's health, well-being, and development. Excess weight at an early age can hinder movement and promote weight gain. It can also affect future health.

To learn more about the need to fight obesity in the early years of your child's life, see:

http://www.youtube.com/watch?v=0HP4i9yw3pA&feature=player_detailpage

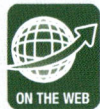

Approximately 10% of children less than two years of age are at or above the 95th percentile of weight-for-length.

15. Is fat but fit a myth?

The answer is yes. Although some obese kids seem healthy, there's no such thing as benign obesity. The unhealthy effects on metabolism start early and can have lifelong effects. Even obese children who are metabolically healthy are more likely to have risk factors for cardiovascular disease, such as high cholesterol or hypertension.

According to the CDC, 70% of obese youth in a population-based sample of children 5–17 years of age had at least one risk factor for cardiovascular disease.

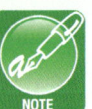

16. Why is it so easy to put on weight and so hard to take it off?

Gaining weight is easy. Losing excess body fat and keeping it off are extremely difficult. This is due in part to genetic factors that influence where we store fat, how fast we eat, and how much fat we burn during physical activity. These genes vary from one child to the next. Scientists are starting to learn how these differences make some kids more prone to obesity.

Gut hormones also play a role: leptin sates hunger, while ghrelin increases appetite. Besides inherent biological and genetic factors, other potential contributors to obesity include aspects of the environment in which we live, such as school, family, social, and cultural interactions. Often these determine whether the healthy food choice is the easy one for parents and children.

Calorie balance is like a scale. To remain in balance and maintain body weight, what children eat must be balanced by the calories they burn in normal body functions, daily activities, and exercise.

PRACTICAL TIP Weight management is all about balancing the number of calories children take in with the number of calories they expend.

DEFINITION A **calorie** is defined as a unit of energy supplied by food. This is so regardless of where it comes from: a candy bar or an apple, carbohydrates, fats, sugars, or protein.

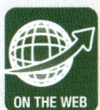

ON THE WEB To learn more about how to balance calorie intake and output, see Video 2.1: Finding Balance.

Calorie balance status.

IF YOU ARE:	YOUR CALORIC-BALANCE STATUS IS:
Maintaining your weight	**In balance:** You are eating roughly the same number of calories that your body is using. Your weight will remain **stable**.
Gaining weight	**In caloric excess:** You are eating more calories than your body is using. You will store these extra calories as fat and will **gain** weight.
Losing weight	In caloric deficit: You are eating fewer calories than you are using. Your body is pulling fat from its storage cells for energy, so your weight will be **decreasing**.

SOURCE: CDC, Healthy Weight

http://www.cdc.gov/healthyweight/calories/index.html

17. What health problems are associated with childhood obesity?

For information on the health effects of childhood obesity, see Video 2.2: Childhood Obesity.

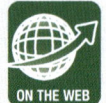

ON THE WEB

The dangers of childhood obesity are many and include serious health risks. We describe some of the more common conditions in the section that follows.

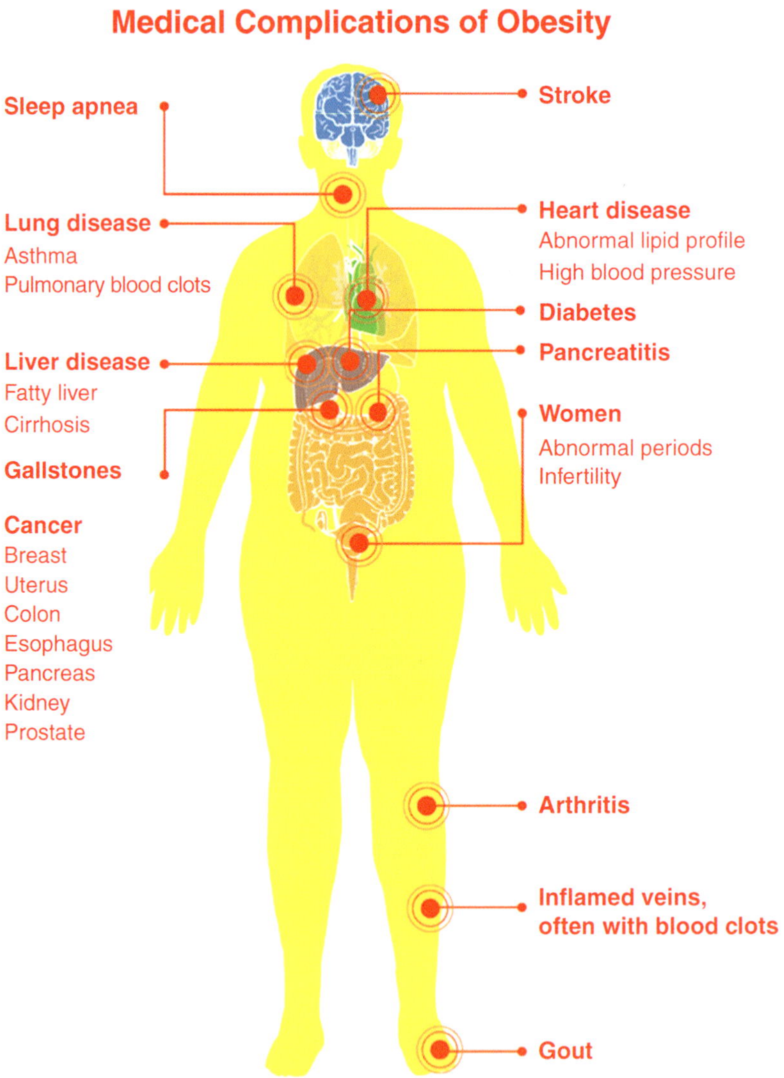

Medical Complications of Obesity
Sleep apnea
Stroke
Lung disease
Asthma
Pulmonary blood clots
Heart disease
Abnormal lipid profile
High blood pressure
Diabetes
Liver disease
Fatty liver
Cirrhosis
Pancreatitis
Gallstones
Women
Abnormal periods
Infertility
Cancer
Breast
Uterus
Colon
Esophagus
Pancreas
Kidney
Prostate
Arthritis
Inflamed veins,
often with blood clots
Gout

FIGURE 2.1
Complications of childhood obesity.

Sleep Problems

Obstructive Sleep Apnea (OSA) can lead to heart disease. Episodes of disturbed sleep can affect the ability to concentrate and perform well in school. They can also cause enuresis (involuntary urination or an inability to control urine flow). OSA is more common among children who are severely obese. Symptoms include loud snoring with pauses in breathing, restless sleep, and daytime sleepiness.

In obesity hypoventilation syndrome, the weight of fat on the chests and abdomens of severely obese children impairs breathing. Symptoms are similar to those of OSA, but treatment requires continuous positive airway pressure (CPAP) until substantial weight loss relieves the condition.

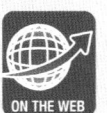

For more information on pediatric sleep apnea, visit:

http://www.entnet.org/HealthInformation/Could-Child-Have-Sleep-Apnea.cfm

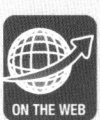

For more information on obesity hypoventilation syndrome, visit:

http://www.nhlbi.nih.gov/health/health-topics/topics/ohs/

To find out more about CPAP, visit:

http://www.entnet.org/HealthInformation/cpap.cfm

Respiratory Problems

Asthma occurs more frequently among obese children. Symptoms might include shortness of breath and exercise intolerance. To minimize limitations on exercise, youngsters may need guidance on how to manage their asthma during physical activity or outdoor play.

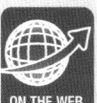

To learn more about asthma, visit:

http://www.nhlbi.nih.gov/health/public/lung/asthma/asthma_atglance.pdf

Gastrointestinal Problems

Nonalcoholic fatty liver disease (NAFLD) is strongly linked to severe obesity in children and adolescents. Defining characteristics are excess abdominal fat and insulin resistance (reduced ability of insulin to lower blood sugar levels). One of the most

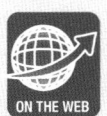

To find out more about NAFLD, visit:

http://www.liverfoundation.org/abouttheliver/info/nafld/

To learn more about gallstones, visit:

http://digestive.niddk.nih.gov/ddiseases/pubs/gallstones/

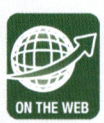

common liver diseases in the U.S. and worldwide, NAFLD can lead to fibrosis, cirrhosis, and may even require liver transplantation. The disease generally has no symptoms, although some patients can have upper right quadrant stomach pain or tenderness, or swelling in the area around the liver. Weight loss leads to improved liver and blood test outcomes.[6]

Gallstones are another intestinal problem among overweight and obese children. Symptoms include episodes of intense colicky pain in the upper right area of the abdomen. Milder stomach pain can also occur. Other common pediatric gastrointestinal problems made worse by obesity include gastroesophageal reflux disease (heartburn) and constipation.

Endocrine Disorders

To find out more about insulin resistance, visit:

http://www.joslin.org/info/what_is_insulin_resistance.html

To learn more about glucose intolerance, go to:

http://www.joslin.org/info/diagnosing_impaired_glucose_tolerance_IGT.html

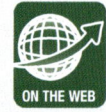

Type 2 diabetes is characterized by high levels of glucose in the blood due to defects in insulin production, the body's ability to use insulin to reduce blood sugar, or both. Serious long-term complications can lead to amputations and premature death. Type 2 diabtes can damage the cardiovascular system, kidneys, eyes, nerves, blood vessels, skin, gums, and teeth. Obese school-aged children and adolescents have adverse changes in the structure and function of their circulatory system, including increased arterial stiffness.[7] Impaired glucose tolerance, a strong predictor of future development of type 2 diabetes, is widespread among children and adolescents with severe obesity. Insulin resistance is the most important factor in the development of impaired glucose tolerance.

To learn more about diabetes, visit:

http://www.youtube.com/watch?v=MGL6km1NBWE

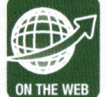

Children and adolescents diagnosed with type 2 diabetes are generally obese, between 10 and 19 years old, and have a strong family history of type 2 diabetes and insulin resistance.

Obese children with early puberty start to physically mature sooner than normal-weight kids. Those at risk are white girls up to seven years old, black girls six years old or younger with breast tissue or pubic hair, and boys younger than nine years with pubic hair or enlargement of the penis.

Polycystic ovary syndrome (PCOS) most often affects obese women 18–25 years of age. It's characterized by excess hairiness, acne, and acanthosis nigricans (see below). Women with PCOS often have insulin resistance or type 2 diabetes and may have metabolic syndrome (a cluster of risk factors that leads to cardiovascular disease).

Skin Conditions

Acanthosis nigricans is a skin disorder in which there is darker, thick, velvety skin in body folds and creases. It is most often found in black children with obesity-related insulin resistance, but it can also occur in obese white youngsters. It usually appears slowly. Symptoms include very visible markings and creases in the armpits, groin, and neck folds, and over the joints of the fingers and toes. Less commonly, the lips, palms, soles of the feet, or other areas may be affected.

Cardiovascular Risk Factors

Cardiovascular risk factors in children and adolescents include high BMI and other measures of body fat, hypertension (blood pressure of more than 140/90 mmHg), and elevated lipids (fats in the blood) and lipoproteins (cholesterol). Insulin resistance, signs of inflammation (an indicator of cardiovascular disease risk), and adverse changes in the structure and function of veins and arteries are other risk factors. The more severe the obesity, the greater the number of risk factors, and the worse the cardiovascular risk profile; for example, high levels of low-density lipoprotein (LDL cholesterol) can be a harbinger of early atherosclerosis or fatty deposits in coronary arteries. These abnormalities in youth may have an effect on later cardiac health.[7]

 In a population-based sample of children and adolescents 5–17 years of age, 70% of obese youth had at least one risk factor for cardiovascular disease.

Lipid abnormalities can become cardiovascular disease risk factors. Cholesterol and triglycerides are lipids or fats that are

Acceptable, borderline, high, and abnormal pediatric lipid levels.

	TOTAL CHOLESTEROL LEVELS	LOW-DENSITY LIPOPROTEIN LEVELS ("BAD" CHOLESTEROL)	TRIGLYCERIDE LEVELS	HIGH-DENSITY LIPOPROTEIN LEVELS ("GOOD" CHOLESTEROL)
Acceptable	< 170 mg/dL	< 110 mg/dL		
Borderline	170–199 mg/dL	110–129 mg/dL		
High	≥ 200 mg/dL	≥ 130 mg/dL		
Abnormal			≥ 110 mg/dL for adolescents	≤ 40 mg/dL for adolescents

SOURCE: Based on U.S. Preventive Services Task Force recommendations.[6]

≥ means equal to or greater than, ≤ means equal to or less than, < means less than

To learn about the effect of high triglyceride levels on a child's life, see Video 2.5: Maya's story.

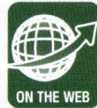
ON THE WEB

To find out more about cholesterol, visit:

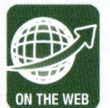
ON THE WEB

http://www.medicinenet.com/cholesterol_management/article.htm

To find out more about triglycerides, visit:

http://www.medicinenet.com/triglyceride_test/article.htm

In general, children who have metabolic syndrome are twice as likely to suffer from heart disease and five times as likely to develop diabetes compared with those who don't have it.

NOTE

easily stored in the body. A source of fuel, they're an important part of the structure of cells. However, when lipid levels are abnormal, they put cardiovascular health at risk. Dyslipidemia is among the most common obesity-related medical conditions in obese children.[6]

Metabolic syndrome is a clustering of conditions that place a child at high risk for heart disease. These include a large waistline (or abdominal obesity), low high-density lipoprotein levels (HDL cholesterol) that can raise the risk for heart problems, elevated fasting blood sugar and triglyceride levels, and hypertension, which can eventually damage the heart and lead to a buildup of plaque in the arteries.

All of these are associated with elevated blood insulin levels. Drugs that decrease insulin resistance and lower blood pressure improve lipid profiles.

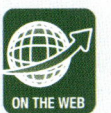 To learn more about metabolic syndrome, visit:

http://www.nhlbi.nih.gov/health/health-topics/topics/ms/

Orthopedic Disorders

Overweight and obese youth suffer more musculoskeletal problems than their normal-weight peers. These include hip and/or knee pain, higher rates of fractures, a higher rate of misalignment in their lower extremities, and reduced ability to walk, run, or play. Another possible problem is a growth disorder, Blount's disease. It is a usually painless bowing of the legs that typically occurs after eight years of age.[6,7] Injury and pain interfere with physical activity, making early intervention (including physical therapy) important to reduce weight gain.

18. What psychosocial problems are associated with childhood obesity?

Obesity can have pronounced effects on quality of life for severely obese children and adolescents. Depression is common, as are emotional and social problems. Poor academic performance is typical. Eating disorders (binge eating and loss of control) are also prevalent.[7] Obese children are

 More than 44% of current and past bullying victims are at "the lowest one-tenth of psychosocial health."
— Laura M. Bogart, PhD, associate professor of pediatrics, Harvard Medical School

often the target of bullies; their abuse can have serious long-term effects on physical and mental health. In addition, obese children have more diagnoses of attention deficit hyperactivity disorder (ADHD) than their slimmer peers. Symptoms include hyperactivity and problems staying focused, paying attention, and controlling behavior.[8]

19. Does childhood obesity affect school attendance?

While there are many reasons for school absenteeism, childhood obesity is a very common one. A study on the attendance patterns of fourth, fifth, and sixth graders in Philadelphia found that obese children were out of school more often than their average-weight counterparts.

 In 2013, obese adolescents had 37% more sick days than their normal-weight counterparts.[10]

This loss of school days can lead to poor grades, missed work for parents, and high costs for school systems.[9]

20. Can obesity in childhood affect adult health?

To find out more about athero-sclerosis, visit:

https://www.nhlbi.nih.gov/health/health-topics/topics/atherosclerosis/

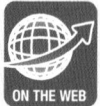

ON THE WEB

Obese children and adolescents are more likely to become obese adults, with risk factors persisting over time. In later years, they typically have adverse levels of cardiovascular and metabolic risk factors. These include insulin resistance, high blood pressure, and elevated lipids (triglycerides) and liver-function enzymes. Severely obese adolescents are also at greater risk of metabolic syndrome. Inflammation (for example, C-reactive protein) follows obese children and adolescents into adulthood, leading to higher levels of oxidized LDL cholesterol (or cholesterol that's been modified by a reaction with oxygen). This is the final step before the development of atherosclerosis.[7]

A more extensive list of obesity-related adult diseases includes:

- Coronary heart disease
- Type 2 diabetes
- Many types of cancers, including those of the breast, colon, endometrium, esophagus, kidney, pancreas, gallbladder, thyroid, ovary, cervix, and prostate, as well as multiple myeloma and Hodgkin's lymphoma
- Hypertension (high blood pressure)
- Dyslipidemia (for example, high LDL cholesterol or triglycerides)
- Stroke
- Liver and gallbladder disease
- Sleep apnea and breathing problems
- Osteoarthritis (a breakdown of cartilage and bone within a joint)
- Gynecological problems, such as abnormal menstrual periods or infertility.

To find out more about the physiological, psychological, and social consequences of obesity, visit:

http://frac.org/initiatives/hunger-and-obesity/what-are-the-consequences-of-adult-overweight-and-obesity/

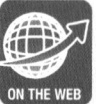

ON THE WEB

In adults, obesity is defined as a BMI of 30 kg/m² or higher. Severe obesity is defined as a BMI of 40 kg/m² or higher.

Risk Assessment for Childhood Obesity

21. What are some common misperceptions about excess weight in infants and children?

Even if excess weight may not yet be apparent, unusually rapid growth in infant weight-for-length puts a child at risk for obesity.[11] It behooves parents to be aware of risk factors for early overweight or obesity in their children. It's never okay for babies to be chubby; even if children are genetically prone to be obese, it doesn't have to be their destiny. More often than not, parents can see obesity in unrelated children but underestimate it in their own.

Infants with high birth weight who gain pounds rapidly in their first four months of life are at risk for later obesity in childhood.

22. What factors increase the risk of obesity in children?

Cheap, delicious, high calorie foods targeted specifically to boys and girls are one of the main drivers of the obesity epidemic. However, knowing a child's risk factors can help offset the negative impact of our obesogenic environment. In this section, we cover some of the most important risk factors for childhood obesity.

High Birth Weight and Appetite

Assessment of weight pattern at birth is important. Higher birth weight (more than 8.8 pounds) and a hearty appetite in early infancy are risk factors for rapid growth. Kids who want second helpings and extra desserts are more likely to become obese as they get older. Normal weight gain, which is fast in the first year of life, is followed

Children who are obese when they enter kindergarten have about a 50% chance of being obese by eighth grade.

by slower growth that reaches a first maximum at the age of 12 months, and then declines. While normal-weight children reach the 12-month maximum BMI again between the ages of nine and ten, overweight and obese children get there much earlier (five to seven years of age).

Very Low Birth Weight

Very low and very high birth weights are both associated with childhood obesity. Catch-up growth may be the link between low birth weight and obesity. Babies who are deprived of nutrition before birth may be primed for fast growth after birth when exposed to a rich nutrient environment (usually infant formula). This rapid growth in the first few months, if not the first days of postnatal life, is associated with an increased risk of being an obese child.[12]

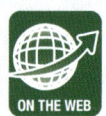

To learn more about birth weight, visit:

http://www.nlm.nih.gov/medlineplus/birthweight.html

ON THE WEB

Parental Weight

How much parents weigh is a major factor in childhood obesity. High BMI is particularly important for several reasons, including shared genes, a common obesogenic lifestyle, and a process called early programming. Early programming refers to nutrition and lifestyle during pregnancy and infancy that can affect a range of body functions, especially those most likely to increase the odds of childhood obesity. Losing weight can help prevent this and lead to improved health for both children and parents.

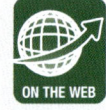

To learn more about the effect of parental obesity on children, visit:

http://www.urmc.rochester.edu/encyclopedia/content.aspx?ContentTypeID=1&ContentID=713

ON THE WEB

Two-year-old children with an insecure attachment pattern are at increased risk for obesity at around four to five years of age.

NOTE

Attachment Patterns

Children with a secure attachment pattern are more easily comforted in stressful situations and better able to regulate negative emotions. This makes them less likely to eat in response to emotional distress in early childhood, when systems in the brain that regulate emotion and appetite are developing at the same time.[13]

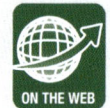

To learn more about early mother-child attachment and obesity, visit:

http://pediatrics.aappublications.org/content/129/1/132.full.pdf

ON THE WEB

Abnormal Adiposity Rebound

Adiposity rebound, the rise in BMI that happens at around six years of age, predicts later body weight. Children with low or normal BMI, followed by a very early adiposity rebound with an increase in body fat, are more likely to be obese and suffer the adverse health effects from the disease (see Chapter 1).

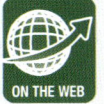

For additional information on BMI rebound and childhood obesity, see Video 3.1: Obesity Rebound.

Sleep

Time spent sleeping plays a key role in preventing obesity. Children who sleep less than 10.5 hours a night at age three have a 45% higher risk of being obese by age seven than their peers who get more than 12 hours of sleep a night. Infants who average less than 12 hours of sleep a day have twice the odds of being obese at age three than those who sleep 12 hours or more. Maternal depression during pregnancy, introduction of solid foods before the age of four months, and TV watching by infants have all been associated with shorter sleep times.[14]

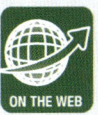

To learn more about the relation between sleep and childhood obesity, visit:

http://www.webmd.com/children/news/20080102/lack-sleep-tied-child-hood-obesity

23. How do prenatal factors influence childhood obesity?

Early life influences, starting with the intrauterine environment and continuing through the first few years of life, shape weight gain and body fatness throughout childhood and adolescence. A number of possible biological pathways link a mother's prepregnancy and prenatal status to obesity in her offspring.

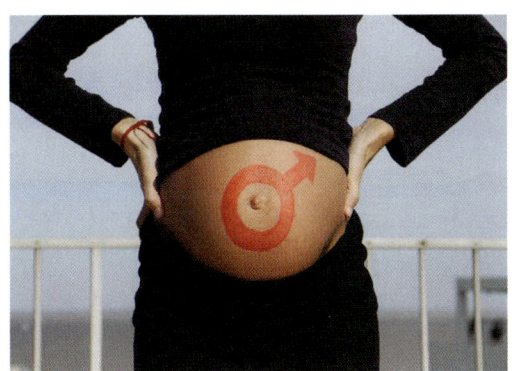

◄ FIGURE 3.1
Prevention of childhood obesity starts before birth. © Naoll

Four factors, in particular, are important in assessing a child's risk for obesity.

Prepregnancy Weight

Women at a higher weight at the onset of pregnancy have infants and children who are more likely to be obese; moreover, the more obese the mother, the greater the effect on her children. Maternal obesity predicts childhood obesity in general, but predicts it most strongly in the more extreme cases. This relationship is apparent in kids under age five as well as in older children and adolescents. The odds are higher that infants of overweight mothers will be born large for gestational age, be less likely to breastfeed (see below), and be at higher risk for obesity and type 2 diabetes later in life.

To learn more about the effects of prepregnancy weight on childhood obesity, visit:

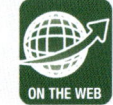
ON THE WEB

http://www.nih.gov/news/pr/dec2005/ninr-05.htm

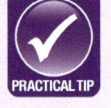
PRACTICAL TIP

Once pregnant, weight loss is not recommended. Having a healthy BMI before pregnancy starts is one of the most important goals for preventing obesity across generations.

Gestational Weight Gain

Gestational weight gain is an independent risk factor for obesity in children and adolescents. Excessive weight gain during pregnancy is relatively common, with more women starting out overweight or obese. Children of those who gain an "excessive" amount of weight have more than four times the risk of being overweight at age three than those whose mothers gain an "inadequate" amount of weight. New guidelines from the Institute of Medicine advocate more moderate weight gain during pregnancy for women who are obese.[11]

Women with a prepregnancy BMI in the normal range (18.5 to 24.9) should gain 25–35 pounds; those with a BMI between 25 and 29.9 should put on only 15–25 pounds. Women with a BMI of 30 or higher should gain only 11–20 pounds.[14]

High maternal weight gain during pregnancy can lead to excess weight retained after childbirth. A high postpartum BMI can be a health risk for mothers by setting the stage for even more excess weight in future pregnancies.

Gestational Diabetes

A mother's gestational diabetes may contribute to obesity in her child. Weight gain during pregnancy is mostly fat tissue. In mid-pregnancy, this excess fat can lead to a state of insulin resistance, an adaptive response that allows more efficient transfer of glucose and other fuels across the placenta to help the fetus grow. However, it may also expose a fetus to periods of high blood glucose and elevated insulin. This can increase birth weight, which is directly associated with later BMI.

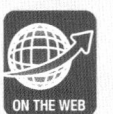

To find out more about gestational diabetes, visit:

http://www.diabetes.org/diabetes-basics/gestational/

Smoking During Pregnancy

Although smoking can help keep off adult weight under ordinary circumstances, doing so during pregnancy can have the opposite effect on the developing fetus. Maternal smoking during pregnancy is associated with a 500% greater risk of obesity at age five and a 260% greater risk at ages nine to ten. The duration of smoking while pregnant and the number of cigarettes smoked per day are both linked to increased rates of childhood obesity. Maternal smoking can lead to low intrauterine growth as well as changes in the volume of the amygdala, the brain's reward center. Both can result in accelerated postnatal growth and childhood obesity.

24. What postnatal factors influence childhood obesity?

Cesarean Delivery

The odds of obesity in children delivered by cesarean section (C-section) double by three years of age compared with infants born vaginally. One possible reason is that a C-section birth might change gut bacteria that affect the way food is digested. Also, mothers who deliver by C-section tend to weigh more than those who deliver vaginally. High maternal weight is a recognized risk factor for childhood obesity.

Breastfeeding

Breastfeeding helps protect against childhood obesity. A baby's risk of becoming overweight falls with each week of breastfeeding.

Breastfeeding for nine months reduces a baby's odds of becoming overweight by more than 30%.

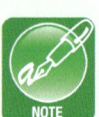

While 75% of mothers start out breastfeeding, only 13% of babies are exclusively breastfed at the end of six months.

For nearly all infants, it is the best source of nutrition and immunologic protection. It also provides many health benefits to mothers (see Chapter 4).

The protective effect of breastfeeding most likely results from a combination of factors that differentiate it from infant formula. The latter contains nearly double the amount of protein per serving as breast milk, an increase that may stimulate unhealthy insulin secretion. Babies also have a different biological response to breast milk than they do to formula, which increases concentrations of insulin in the blood and prolongs insulin response. Even into childhood, formula is associated with reduced leptin, a hormone that holds appetite in check and controls body fatness.[12]

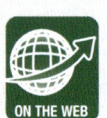

Phthalates are a type of hormone disruptor used in plastics (most often PVC) and in personal care products. Significantly higher levels have been found in the bodies of overweight young girls than in the general population of children.

To learn more about chemical exposure and obesity, visit:

http://www.ncbi.nlm.nih.gov/pmc/articles/PMC3279464/

Chemical Exposures

Fetal and infant exposure to endocrine disrupting chemicals or "obesogens" may promote obesity by increasing the number of fat cells, changing the amount of calories burned at rest, and altering energy balance and the body's mechanisms for appetite and satiety. It may also lead to more weight gain per calories consumed as well as less weight loss per amount of energy expended. One way exposure can happen is when parents microwave baby bottles or plastic containers not explicitly designated as safe for microwaving.[12]

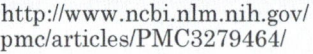

25. What is portion distortion?

Portion sizes of less healthy foods and beverages have increased over time in restaurants, grocery stores, and vending machines. Children served larger portions eat more without realizing it; this adds up to a lot of extra calories, especially with rich desserts and other fattening foods. Average portion sizes have grown radically over the past 20 years. Sometimes there's enough food on a plate for two or more people. Growing portions are changing what Americans think of as a "normal" serving size at home as well. This is portion distortion.

Check out the table below to see examples of how larger portions lead to added calories:

Portion sizes 20 years ago and today.

	20 YEARS AGO		TODAY	
	PORTION	CALORIES	PORTION	CALORIES
Bagel	3-inch diameter	140	6-inch diameter	350
Cheeseburger	1	333	1	590
Spaghetti with meatballs	1 cup sauce 3 small meatballs	500	2 cups sauce 3 large meatballs	1,020
Soda	6.5 ounces	82	20 ounces	250
Blueberry muffin	1.5 ounces	210	5 ounces	500

SOURCE: National Heart, Lung, and Blood Institute, Serving Sizes and Portions

https://www.nhlbi.nih.gov/health/public/heart/obesity/wecan/eat-right/distortion.htm

It can be hard to eat or drink a healthy portion size. Many people don't even know what one is anymore. Restaurants typically serve large meals, and the food and beverage industries use super-sized packaging to sell more products.

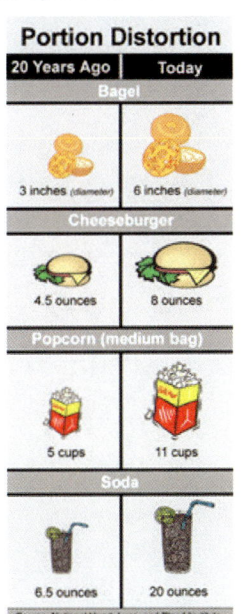

Portion Distortion

20 Years Ago	Today
Bagel	
3 inches (diameter)	6 inches (diameter)
Cheeseburger	
4.5 ounces	8 ounces
Popcorn (medium bag)	
5 cups	11 cups
Soda	
6.5 ounces	20 ounces

Source: National Heart, Lung, and Blood Institute

➤ **FIGURE 3.2**
Portion distortion over time

The following material comes largely from the CDC's "A Growing Problem." It can be found at

http://www.cdc.gov/obesity/childhood/problem.html

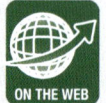

Sugary Drinks

Sugary drinks and less healthy foods on school campuses affect some 55 million school-aged children. Even though sugar-sweetened beverages and high-fat snacks contribute to obesity, more than half of U.S. middle and high schools still sell them. Children can have them just about any time they want. They're readily available through vending machines, school canteens, sporting events, and fundraising and other parties.

Multimillion Dollar Advertising Campaigns

Major advertising and marketing campaigns by the food and beverage industry promote sales of high-fat, high-calorie foods and snacks to children and teens. Close to half of U.S. middle

In 2009, food and beverage companies spent $149 million on in-school marketing alone.[15]

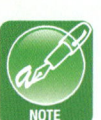

and high schools allow this kind of advertising. It has a powerful and unhealthy influence on young people. In comparison, promotion of healthy foods is almost nonexistent.

Varied Licensing Requirements for Childcare Centers

More than 12 million children spend time in childcare arrangements outside the home. However, not all facilities are licensed based on their ability to provide healthy eating and physical activity.

Lack of Daily High Quality Physical Activity in Schools

To see the *2008 Physical Activity Guidelines for Americans,* visit:

http://www.health.gov/paguidelines

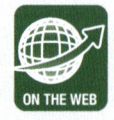

The *2008 Physical Activity Guidelines for Americans* recommends at least 60 minutes of aerobic activity each day for adolescents. Most fall short of this goal. In 2007, only 18% of students in grades 9–12 met the standard; in 2009, only 33% attended daily physical activity classes.

For a youth physical activity guidelines toolkit, visit:

http://www.cdc.gov/healthyyouth/physicalactivity/guidelines.htm

No Safe, Nearby, or Appealing Places to Play or Be Active

In many communities, places for physical activity may be dangerous or hard to find. Parks and recreation centers could be far from home, and public transportation may be unavailable. Many children have no safe routes for walking or biking to a playground. Half of the kids in the U.S. don't have parks, community centers, or sidewalks in their neighborhoods. Only 27 states have policies on community-scale design.

Limited Access to Healthy Affordable Foods

Fast-food restaurants, convenience stores, and other purveyors of cheap, tasty, high-calorie foods and snacks tend to cluster in minority and lower-income neighborhoods. Such areas typically have less access to stores and supermarkets that sell healthy foods at a reasonable price. People who live in rural areas may also be far away from a supermarket. Limited access to affordable fruits and vegetables is associated with increased risk for obesity.

Greater Availability of Energy-Dense Foods and Sugary Drinks

Energy-dense foods have a lot of calories in each bite. A diet with too many of these foods causes excess body fat in children. Sugary drinks are the biggest culprit. They have few, if any, nutrients, yet account for a high number of calories in the diets of U.S. youngsters. On a typical day, 80% of children and adolescents drink sugary beverages.

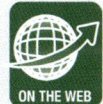

To see a sugary drink and obesity fact sheet, visit:

http://www.hsph.harvard.edu/nutritionsource/sugary-drinks-fact-sheet/

27. What is screen time?

Screen time is the number of hours spent using entertainment media, including television or movies, DVDs, video or computer games, the Internet, texting, Facebook, and other social media.

On average, children younger than two years of age watch television 1–2 hours a day. By the time they're three years old, almost 33% of children have a television in their bedroom. Youth aged 8–18 spend over 7.5 hours a day watching TV and movies, sitting in front of computers (not doing homework), playing video games, or using cell phones.[14]

To learn more about the pros and cons of screen time, visit:

https://www.youtube.com/watch?v=_pPNuRMQ5QI

ON THE WEB

These sedentary pursuits take up time that could be spent playing sports or taking part in other physical activities. They lead to increased snacking and eating meals in front of the TV, while food and beverage ads entice them to make unhealthy food choices.

References and Endnotes

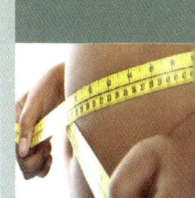

CHAPTER 1

1. World Health Organization. (2015). *Childhood Overweight and Obesity*. Global Strategy of Diet, Physical Activity and Health. Available at: http://www.who.int/dietphysicalactivity/childhood/en/. Accessed February 10, 2014.

2. Tavernise S. (2014). *Obesity Rate for Young Children Plummets 43% in a Decade*. Available at: http://www.nytimes .com/2014/02/26/health/obesity-rate-for-young-children-plummets-43-in-a-decade.html?action=click&contentCollection=U.S.&region =Footer&module=TopNews&pgtype. Accessed February 27, 2014.

3. Ogden C.L., Carroll M.D., Kit B.K., et al. (2014). *Prevalence of Childhood and Adult Obesity in the United States, 2011-2012*. JAMA, 311: 806-814.

4. Wang Y.C., Gortmaker S.L., Sobol A.M., et al. (2006). *Estimating the Energy Gap Among U.S. Children: A Counterfactual Approach*. Pediatrics, 118:e 1721-1733.

5. World Health Organization. (2015). *Child Growth Standards*. The WHO Child Growth Standards. Available at: http://www.who.int/childgrowth/standards/en/. Accessed February 10, 2014.

CHAPTER 2

6. US Preventive Services Task Force, Barton M. (2010). *Screening for obesity in children and adolescents: U.S. Preventive Services Task Force recommendation statement*. Pediatrics, 125(2): 361-367.

7. Kelly A.S., Barlow S.E., Rao G., et al. (2013). *Severe Obesity in Children and Adolescents: Identification, Associated Health Risks, and Treatment Approaches: A Scientific Statement from the American Heart Association*. Circulation, 128(15): 1689-1712.

8. Pulgaron E.R. (2013). *Childhood Obesity: A Review of Increased Risk for Physical and Psychological Comorbidities*. Clin Ther, 35(1): A18-32.

9. Geier A.B., Foster G.D., Womble L.G., et al. (2007). *The Relationship Between Relative Weight and School Attendance Among Elementary Schoolchildren*. Obesity, 15(8): 2157-2161.

10. Pan L., Sherry B., Park S., Blanck H.M. (2009). *The Association of Obesity and School Absenteeism Attributed to Illness or Injury Among Adolescents in the United States*. J Adolesc Health, 52(1): 64-69.

11. Committee on Obesity Prevention Policies for Young Children. Birch LL, Parker L, Burns A, Editors. (2015). *Early Childhood Obesity Prevention Policies.* Institute of Medicine of the National Academies, Washington, D.C. Available at: http://books.nap.edu/ openbook.php?record_id=13124. Accessed February 12, 2015.

12. White House Task Force on Childhood Obesity. (2010). *Solving the Problem of Childhood Obesity Within a Generation.* Report to the President. Available at: http://www.letsmove.gov/sites/lets-move.gov/files/TaskForce_on_Childhood_Obesity_May2010_Full-Report.pdf. Accessed March 18, 2014.

13. Anderson S.E., Whitaker R.C. (2011). *Attachment Security and Obesity in U.S. Preschool-Aged Children.* Arch Pediatr Adolesc Med. 165(3): 235-242.

14. *Obesity Prevention Source.* Harvard School of Public Health. Available at: http://www.hsph.harvard.edu/obesity-prevention-source/obesity-causes/sleep-and-obesity/. Accessed March 18, 2014.

15. Harris J.L., Fox T. (2014). *Food and Beverage Marketing in Schools: Putting Student Health at the Head of the Class.* JAMA Pediatr, 168(3): 206-208.

PART TWO

PREVENTING CHILDHOOD OBESITY

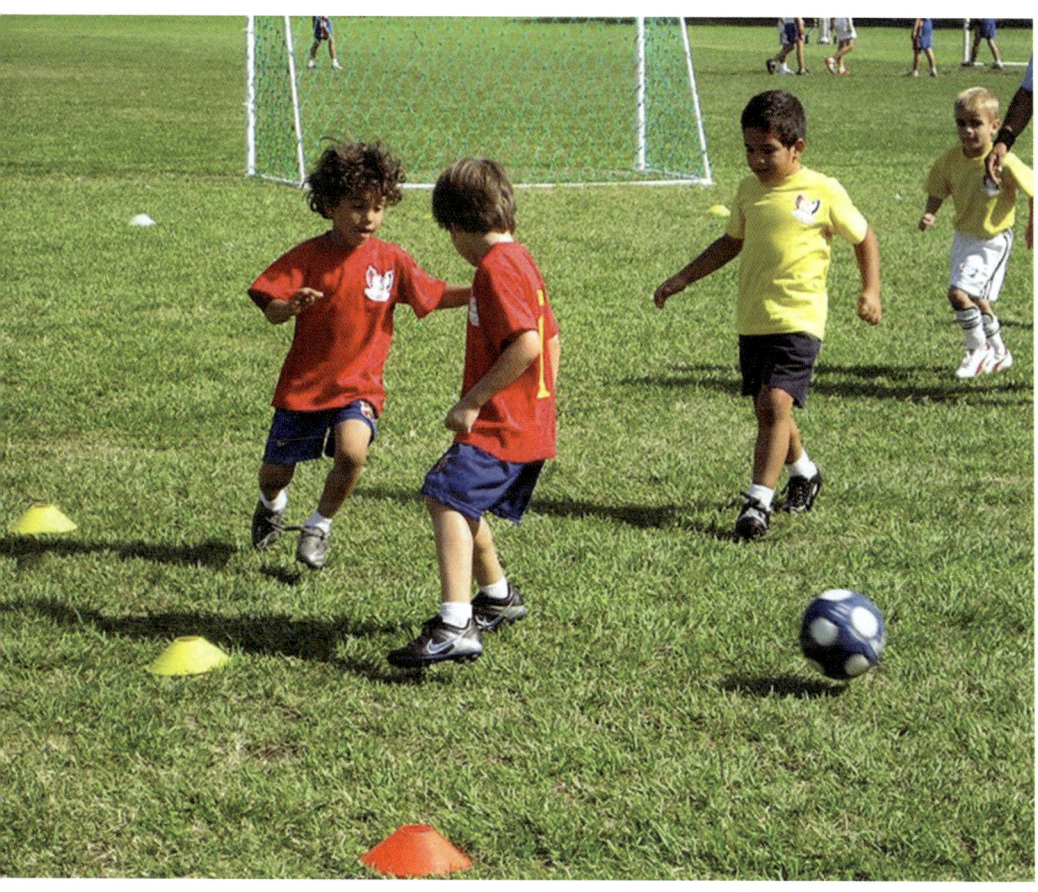

In Part Two, we define prevention of childhood obesity and discuss why it's important to stop the disease before it starts. We describe the differences between prevention and intervention, and cover what, how, and when to feed infants, toddlers, and preschoolers to promote healthy and active living. We discuss the joys and challenges of breastfeeding and the best ways to bottle feed. We also talk about the need for adequate sleep and physical activity at each growth stage and discuss steps parents can take to teach healthy living from childhood through young adulthood.

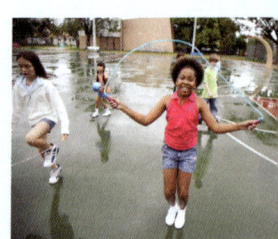

CHAPTER 4
Preventing Obesity in Infants

CHAPTER 5
Preventing Obesity in Toddlers

CHAPTER 6
Preventing Obesity in Preschoolers

CHAPTER 7
Preventing Obesity in Middle Childhood

CHAPTER 8
Preventing Obesity in Adolescence

Preventing Obesity in Infants (0 to 12 Months)

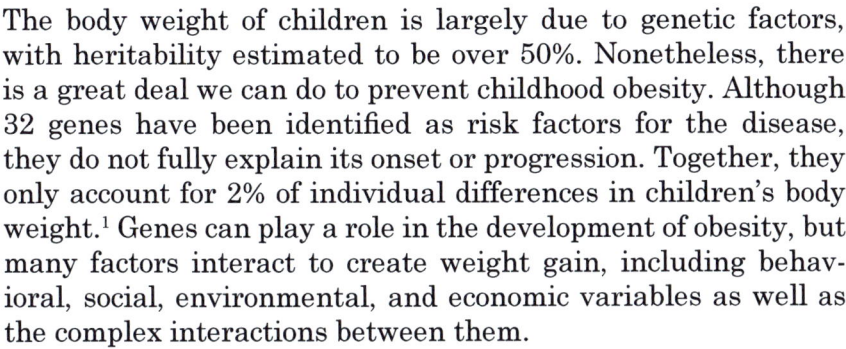

28. Can obesity be prevented?

The body weight of children is largely due to genetic factors, with heritability estimated to be over 50%. Nonetheless, there is a great deal we can do to prevent childhood obesity. Although 32 genes have been identified as risk factors for the disease, they do not fully explain its onset or progression. Together, they only account for 2% of individual differences in children's body weight.[1] Genes can play a role in the development of obesity, but many factors interact to create weight gain, including behavioral, social, environmental, and economic variables as well as the complex interactions between them.

29. What's the difference between prevention and intervention?

Two kinds of interventions are used to fight childhood obesity. Those for primary prevention are designed to keep children who aren't overweight or obese from ever becoming so. They largely address risk factors that could promote positive energy balance, such as not having safe and adequate playgrounds nearby, or a lack of knowledge on how to create a healthy food environment.

Weight loss interventions usually aim to help children lose weight, and for the most part, work to modify diet, physical activity, or sedentary behavior. Although not intended to achieve weight loss, prevention programs that include all children in a population may also help those who are obese lose or stabilize weight.

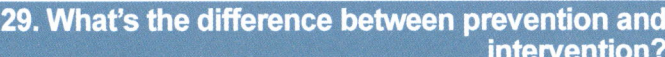

...evention is the act of stopping something from happening or arising.
...tervention is action taken ...improve a situation, especially a ...dical disorder.

DEFINITION

30. How early should prevention begin?

As with any disease, prevention is easier than treatment. This is especially true with obesity: if your child is obese when he or she enters kindergarten, odds are that obesity and its associated health problems will carry over to adulthood. It's critically important to prevent the disease during the early years. Ideally, prevention should start before pregnancy (see Chapter 3) and continue through infancy, toddlerhood, and the preschool years.[2]

31. What factors are most important in preventing obesity in infants (0–12 months)?

A number of factors affect prevention of obesity in infants, including:

- what, when, and how much you feed your infant
- the strength of bonding between mother and child
- whether an infant gets enough of the right kinds of physical activity
- whether your infant sleeps enough during the first few years of his or her life

32. Should I breastfeed?

Many parents are surprised to find out that babies who are breastfed for at least six months are less likely to be overweight or obese as they get older. Breastfeeding helps protect against childhood obesity and other illnesses. The American Academy of Pediatrics recommends exclusive breastfeeding for the first six months of an infant's life, with continued breastfeeding for at least one year. Breastfeeding can be hard work, but it's an excellent way to bond with your baby and help him or her stay healthy.[2]

The best way to get started with breastfeeding is to set small goals:
- plan to breastfeed for the next two weeks instead of the next six months
- ask for support from your partner and family
- ask other women who've breastfed their babies what worked best for them

PRACTICAL TIP

33. What are some problems I might encounter if I breastfeed?

It's normal for moms who breastfeed for the first time to worry about:

- whether the baby is getting enough milk
- if the baby has latched onto the nipple the right way

- pain in the breast or nipple
- spending what seems to be all their time breastfeeding

For about the first month, babies usually need to breastfeed every two to three hours. In time, their stomachs can hold more, and they nurse less often. It's important to respond quickly to signals that your baby is full; for example, if he or she turns her head away or falls asleep. Encouraging an infant to eat more than what he or she needs can disrupt natural appetite-satiety mechanisms. Babies instinctively know when to start and stop feeding.

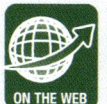

Latching on to the nipple properly is particularly important for the well-being of mother and infant. To learn about tips for breastfeeding, visit:

http://www.youtube.com/watch?v-=IS1XuKbJ0yg

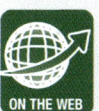

For a more in-depth look at common breastfeeding problems, visit:

http://www.uptodate.com/contents/common-breastfeeding-problems-beyond-the-basics

34. Where can I get help with breastfeeding?

Your doctor or child's pediatrician can help guide you through the process of learning how to breastfeed. Sometimes hospitals also have resources you can tap into. In addition, most insurance plans will pay for you to speak to a breastfeeding expert.

Lactation consultants are also playing an increasingly important role in helping breastfeeding women and their families. The International Lactation Consultant Association (ILCA) is the professional organization for Board Certified Lactation Consultants®.

ILCA has more than 6,000 members from over 80 nations including board-certified lactation consultants, midwives, nurses, physicians, childbirth educators, dietitians, support counselors, and other healthcare professionals.

Breastfeeding may look easy and natural to observers, but it's not simple. New moms

To find out where you can find a nearby lactation consultant, visit:

http://www.ilca.org/i4a/pages/index.cfm?pageid=3337

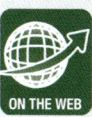

To watch a lactation consultant help a new mom learn how to breastfeed her baby, see Video 4.1: 10 Tips for Breastfeeding Success have much to learn, including key breastfeeding positions, what to do about sore nipples, and other common nursing challenges. These can run the gamut from an infection called mastitis (a breast infection with flu-like symptoms) to thrush (a fungal infection).

One place to get comprehensive breastfeeding support is from the La Leche League. For more information on what this group has to offer, visit:

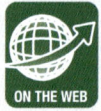
ON THE WEB

http://www.llli.org/resources/assistance.html?m=0,,0.

Every new mother has questions or concerns about breastfeeding, and a growing number of resources are available to help address various issues that might come up. These include 800 numbers for free support and organizations like the La Leche League and KellyMom.

35. What happens if I can't or don't want to breastfeed?

Some mothers can't breastfeed or choose not to do so. If you're among this group, you'll want to know all you can about bottle- and formula-feeding. Baby formula can meet all of your infant's nutritional needs, but like breastfeeding, it requires knowing what to do and how to do it.

For tips on how to start bottle-feeding, visit:

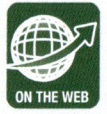
ON THE WEB

http://www.babycenter.com/0_bottle-feeding-basics_752.bc

36. Are all formulas the same?

Most supermarkets carry a baffling array of baby formulas. Some are based on cow's milk, others on soy. Some are iron-fortified, while others are made for babies who are lactose intolerant. Even if you don't know which way to turn when you hit the baby-formula aisle, you can take some comfort in the fact that all formulas made in the United States meet strict FDA guidelines for nutrition. Just don't buy damaged cans or products that have been on the shelves beyond their expiration date.

To find out more about what kinds of formulas are out there and how to choose the best one for your baby, visit:

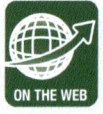
ON THE WEB

http://www.webmd.com/parenting/baby/baby-formula

37. How much should I feed my infant?

At first, give your infant about two ounces of formula every two to three hours. As your baby grows, you'll need to increase the amount of formula. By the end of the first month, he or she should be taking in an average of at least four ounces of formula per feeding. At six months of age, your baby will be consuming six to eight ounces per feeding. In general, you'll be feeding your infant when he or she is hungry, usually five to six times in 24 hours.

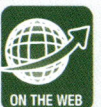

To find out more about how much and how often your baby needs to eat, go to:

http://www.babble.com/baby/babble-formula-feeding-guide/formula-feeding-guide-how-much-when-to-feed/

38. What safety issues are there in bottle-feeding an infant?

When it comes to feeding your baby, there are many more safety issues to consider than just not making the formula too hot or too cool. The rules are iron-clad and include, among others, sterilizing all of your baby's feeding equipment, taking one step at a time when boiling water and preparing the formula, putting your baby in the right position for healthy and comfortable eating, accurately reading your baby's food and feeding signals, and appreciating the differences between ready-made and fresh formula.

Here are just a few bottle-feeding safety tips that can prevent problems:

- If a baby is too young to hold a bottle by him- or herself, make sure someone holds it and takes it away when the infant is done feeding.
- Do not use pillows or other items to prop up a bottle for a baby. These can make it hard to spit out the bottle at the end of feeding, pose a choking hazard, and increase the risk of an ear infection. They can also keep your infant eating after he or she is already full.

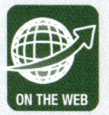

For more detailed instructions on how to safely bottle-feed your baby, visit:

http://www.babycentre.co.uk/a559787/bottle-feeding-your-baby-safely

39. How do I make the move to solid foods?

Although breast milk and formula are the best choices for your baby, he or she will give you signs that it's time to start eating solid food at around four to six months of age. Moving to solid foods (like baby cereal and baby food) is an important part of your baby's development, but starting too early can eventually lead to problems with overweight or obesity.

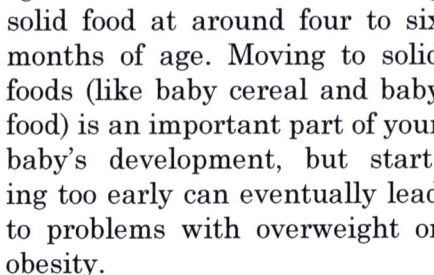

To find out if your baby is ready for solid foods, visit:

http://www.healthychildren.org/English/healthy-living/growing-healthy/Pages/baby-food-and-feeding.aspx#none

ON THE WEB

40. Does my baby need physical activity?

Sometimes parents don't realize that moving and being active are the ways that infants not only learn, but also reach important developmental milestones, like sitting up and crawling. Simple activities will do, such as playing, reaching, grabbing, and having "tummy time" (always with an adult watching); this "playing" helps babies grow into healthy children.

To get your baby moving:
- Invest in a lot of supervised "tummy time." This will make your baby stronger and get him or her ready to sit up and crawl.
- Give your baby many chances to stretch. Use a play mat with toys suspended above him or her. A lot of opportunities to kick and reach will make your baby stronger and also teach him or her about cause and effect.
- Starting around age three or four months, help your baby stand and sit. Do it over and over again until he or she is tired. Make this a fun bonding time for the two of you.

PRACTICAL TIP

Parents should dedicate time every day for active play. A good way to do this is to take five- to ten-minute breaks throughout the day. It's also important to minimize the amount of time babies spend in items that restrict movement (such as car seats, strollers, and bouncy seats). Experts also recommend limiting or eliminating TV, even educational programming. Children who watch more than two hours of TV a day are more likely to be overweight or obese as they get older.[3]

To strengthen your relationship with your infant, do these activities together:

- Read out loud
- Play music and gently dance with him or her in your arms

- Sit and play together on the floor
- Play peekaboo and patty-cake
- Give frequent hugs and loving physical contact

41. How much sleep does my baby need?

Shorter sleep duration and obesity go hand in hand. For newborns less than three months old, the Institute of Medicine recommends sleeping 10.5–18 hours in a 24-hour period.[4] Infants three months to less than twelve months of age should sleep 9–12 hours during the night with 30-minute to 2-hour naps one to four times a day.

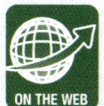

To find out more about how you and your baby can get enough sleep, visit:

http://www.mayoclinic.org/healthy-living/infant-and-toddler-health/in-depth/baby-sleep/art-20045014

Preventing Obesity in Toddlers (12 to 36 Months)

42. Why are toddlers so tough to handle?

Early childhood is a period of rapid physical growth and testing of parental boundaries. Toddlers struggle to be free of their parent's control while unconsciously wanting and needing to be contained and protected. The time between toddlerhood and young childhood is also a period of rapid, cognitive, social, and emotional development.[5]

To help foster healthy active living that prevents overweight and obesity as children grow, a number of desired behaviors are critical. These activities span three broad areas: food and feeding, physical activity, and general parenting. This chapter covers each of them.

Children quadruple their birth weight by age two. Between the ages of two to five years, they gain an average of 4.5–6.5 lbs and grow 2.5–3.5 inches per year.

43. What should I be feeding my child to avoid obesity?

As a parent, you have the vital job of providing a variety of healthy foods every day. For toddlers aged 12 to 24 months, these will include whole milk and other dairy products, iron-fortified cereals, other grains, fruits, vegetables, and protein. For toddlers aged 24 to 36 months, you'll serve the same staples but will switch from whole to low-fat milk and dairy items and add a greater variety of whole grains, fruits, vegetables, and combination foods, such as macaroni and cheese. Ideally, you want your child to eat from each of the basic food groups each day:

1. Meat, fish, poultry, and eggs
2. Milk, cheese, and other dairy products
3. Fruits and vegetables
4. Cereals, potatoes, rice, and flour products

Let your toddler decide what to eat and how much. This will help him or her learn to self-regulate food intake by responding to internal cues of hunger and fullness. By age two, toddlers should be eating three healthy meals a day plus one or two snacks (see Section 46.) They can eat the same food as the rest of the family and use their improved language and social skills to become an active participant at meal times.

To find out more about what and how to feed your toddler, visit:

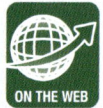

ON THE WEB

http://www.healthychildren.org/English/ healthy-living/growing-healthy/Pages/ toddler-food-and-feeding.aspx#seeAll_8_13

Feeding skills will be more advanced by this time as well. Two year olds are able to use a spoon, drink from a cup with just one hand, and feed themselves with a wide variety of finger foods. As these abilities develop, children switch from eating soft pieces of food to options with more texture. By the ages of three or four, they can use their fingers to push food onto a spoon and pick it up with a fork.

44. What are the best beverages for toddlers?

Low-fat milk or water are the healthiest choices; water is the best between-meal option. Offer whole or 2% milk from 12–24 months of age and low-fat milk after 24 months. These drinks won't get your child used to sweet, sugary tastes. They'll also provide more nutrients and hydration than other drinks and protect teeth by reducing dental decay.

Your child should drink 16 ounces (480 ml) of low-fat or non-fat milk each day. This will provide most of the calcium needed for bone growth without interfering with his or her appetite for other foods. In general, diets rich in low- or nonfat milk and other dairy products are nutritionally sound.[6]

45. Should I let my toddler have flavored milk, juice, or sugar-sweetened beverages as treats?

The answer is no. Juice adds an average of 100 calories a day to a toddler's diet. The same is true for extra calories in sugar-sweetened beverages, including flavored milk. Both drinks can put on unwanted weight and also cause diarrhea, gas, belly bloat, and cavities. If your toddler refuses milk or water, limit juice to 4–6 ounces in a cup and make sure it's 100% juice rather than a juice drink. In a pinch, you can also offer low-fat, low-sugar flavored milk.

 More than half of toddlers and preschoolers consume one or more sugar-sweetened beverages a day.

46. Will snacking lead to obesity?

Snacks aren't treats. Toddlers need two to three healthy snacks a day to satisfy all their nutritional needs; they can't do it with regular meals alone. Fruits and vegetables make for quick and easy options. With a little planning, they can also be ready to go when you're on the run.

Fruits and vegetables are a healthy alternative to prepackaged foods; they provide an opportunity to give your child nutrients. Pediatricians recommend that toddlers eat these snacks at a planned time, while sitting down, and under adult supervision. Don't allow all-day/continuous snacking. It can start your toddler on the path to obesity.

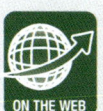 To find out more about healthy fruit and vegetable snacks for toddlers, see Healthy Food Choices: Snacks for Toddlers at:

http://www.youtube.com/watch?v=IRZnAKe5nV4

47. How can I get my child to eat a variety of healthy foods?

Eating only one or two foods or refusing to eat certain kinds of food is normal behavior for toddlers. One way to deal with the picky eater is to offer choices, for example, an apple or banana. This allows your toddler to be independent

 A child might need to try a new food 10–15 times over several months before he or she will eat it.

in a healthy way. Parents provide, children decide: put out a variety of healthy foods every day and let your toddler make his or her choices.

For information on approaches you can use to deal with a picky eater, visit:

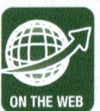

http://www.wholesometoddlerfood.com/

At times, getting your toddler to eat new foods is a matter of preparing the same item in a variety of ways. Other techniques you can use to avoid mealtime battles include letting your child help you prepare healthy meals and snacks, making eating a fun game, or trying certain recipes known to help picky eaters get all the nutrients they need.

To learn more about living with a picky eater, see 19–24 Months Feeding at:

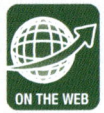

http://www.youtube.com/watch?v=Bsn47f1KXv8

When dealing with picky eaters, remember that you're in charge. Meal time stubbornness is a stage that all toddlers go through; it will pass. In the meantime, relax, present new foods a tablespoon at a time, enjoy your child, be patient, and maintain a sense of humor.

48. How much physical activity does a toddler need to avoid overweight or obesity?

"Play is so important to optimal child development that it has been recognized by the United Nations High Commission for Human Rights as a right of every child." — Dr. Kenneth Ginsburg, Children's Hospital of Philadelphia

The National Association of Sports and Physical Education recommends that children 12–36 months of age get at least 30 minutes of structured adult-led physical activity and 60 minutes to up to several hours per day of unstructured free play. Toddlers shouldn't spend more than one hour being inactive, except when they're sleeping.

Children's play is serious business. Physical activity builds strength, agility, and better coordination. It helps toddlers develop movement skills that are needed for more complex tasks. Kids also learn as they play. They practice making decisions, using their imaginations, building social skills, and becoming leaders.

Play is the time that kids use to explore their world. It helps them process and experience it on their own terms. Unstructured play time is just as important as group or adult-led play. It gives toddlers a chance to be creative, to reflect and relax, and to master their environments.

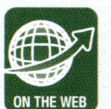

For more information about children's play and the important roles it serves in their lives, see Play is Children's Work:

http://www.youtube.com/watch?v=FR5pO_85fMk

49. My schedule is so hectic, how can I find time to play with my toddler?

Playing together builds strong parent-child bonds and is a critical investment in your toddler's current and future well-being. Structured physical activity is something you plan to do with your toddler. It's the time you carve out of a busy schedule to dance together, play hide-and-seek, or kick a ball around.

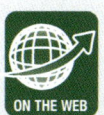

For more ideas on what to do during play time, visit:

http://www.philly.com/philly/blogs/healthy_kids/What-kind-of-physical-activity-does-a-toddler-need.html

50. How do I keep my toddler busy during free-play time?

Toddlers are constantly on the go: crawling, walking, learning to jump, climbing on and off furniture, or pulling toys behind them. By two to three years of age, they run easily and start learning to pedal a tricycle. With their short attention spans, they may jump from one activity to the next, making it hard to keep up with them.

Natural curiosity and energy make free play easy to manage. All you need is an open and safe area, like a playroom, toys or equipment that prompt physical activity, and an adult to supervise (if needed), participate, or help. Toys can be simple and common: a ball, a tricycle or scooter, a few balloons, or blocks. Children's imaginations can also be a good source of ideas for active play, such as pretend housecleaning, vacuuming, sweeping, or raking leaves.

"Play is essential because it contributes to the cognitive, physical, social, and emotional well-being of children and youth." — Dr. Kenneth Ginsburg, Children's Hospital of Philadelphia

51. What should I be looking out for in a childcare setting?

Make sure the facility has plenty of safe and comfortable space for play and a variety of age-appropriate toys. Track your child's activity levels and avoid settings where the television is on all day.

Find out what foods and snacks are available and how they're served. Safety should be a top priority as well. Toddlers should never run around with food in their mouths. To prevent choking, say that you want your child seated while being fed.

52. How much television should I let my toddler watch without increasing the risk of obesity?

A television that's on in child's bedroom for more than two hours a day is a risk factor for being overweight by age three.[7] Kids two years old and younger shouldn't watch any television; those over two should watch less than 120 minutes a day.

If you do let your child watch television:

- Turn on programs that can help your toddler learn important skills, like saying the alphabet and counting
- Turn the TV off during mealtimes, playtime, bath time, and bedtime
- Don't let your child watch entertainment that doesn't stimulate interaction or thought

NOTE

Health care providers also counsel parents and caregivers to keep computers, cell phones, video games, and other hand-held devices out of children's bedrooms or sleep areas. Screen time is a direct competitor for physical activity in kids from birth to 12th grade.

53. Can sleep time affect my toddler's weight?

Being short on sleep can make your toddler cranky. Even worse, it can be the culprit behind early onset obesity. Little kids need a lot of long, solid sleep, at least 12–14 hours a night. Daytime napping doesn't count.

Infants and toddlers in particular are affected by not having enough sleep. In one study, they were more than twice as likely as their well-rested peers to move from a normal weight to overweight or from overweight to obese in a five-year period.[8] Another report found that a seven-year-old child who got less than 12 hours of sleep between the ages of six months and two years had 36% higher odds of being obese than a child who had more sleep during his or her early years.[9]

It could be that kids who don't get enough sleep are too tired to play and run around enough to prevent obesity. Certain hormones, like leptin and ghrelin, might also be to blame. Leptin levels fall in tired kids, telling the body that it needs more food. Meanwhile, levels of ghrelin increase, stimulating the appetite.[8]

Whatever the cause, the message is the same: remove high-tech toys and gadgets from the bedroom at night, be consistent about bedtime, and follow good sleep hygiene practices. Maintain nap routines. Put your child to bed at the same time each night, and tuck him or her in while drowsy but still awake.

At about 15 months of age, some toddlers wake up at night. This is a brief stage. If your child gets up, make a brief, reassuring visit; that's all that's needed. A stuffed animal, blanket, or favorite toy can also help smooth the transition back to sleep.

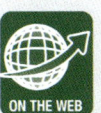

ON THE WEB

To learn more about common toddler sleeping problems and solutions, visit:

http://www.webmd.com/parenting/guide/tackling-toddler-sleep-problems

54. How can I set a good example for my toddler?

Childhood obesity starts at home. Of all the adults who are part of a toddler's life, parents have the greatest influence on habits like eating healthy foods, turning off the television, or getting enough physical activity.

Toddlers copy what you do:

- Eat fruits and vegetables with your child during snack time. The mutual reinforcement will go a long way toward instilling healthy lifelong dietary patterns.
- Show love without food. If your toddler does something commendable, dance around the room together or read a story.
- Make your second helping a vegetable. Small changes in your behavior will be magnified in your child.

55. How do I get other people to support my parenting goals?

Be clear with caregivers. Speak up. Make your wants known. If grandparents show their love by taking your toddler out for ice cream, ask them to go to a park instead. Let them know what your rules are. Give them some alternative ideas. If caregivers don't listen, blame the pediatrician; say the doctor wants your toddler to drink only milk or water. Find out what snacks and meals are served in daycare; make sure that the foods your child eats are available and served in the ways you specify.

56. How do I make the lessons I teach my child about leading a healthy lifestyle stick?

Make the healthy option the easy choice. Establish traditions around good nutrition and physical activity. For example, eat dinner as a family, have breakfast together each morning, serve fruits and vegetables at every meal, and reward your child with a story or a game of hide-and-seek instead of a cookie.

To help your toddler stay at a healthy weight for life, visit:

http://www.healthychildren.org/English/healthy-living/growing-healthy/Pages/assessment.aspx

You bring food into the house. You determine how long your child can watch television. You say when it's time for bed. By and large, you create your toddler's world. Just make sure that it's a healthy, active, and consistent one.

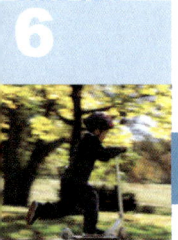

CHAPTER 6

Preventing Obesity in Preschool Children

57. What kinds of changes can I expect to see in my child during the preschool years?

Preschool is a time of developmental milestones for your child. With seemingly boundless energy and drive, he or she will make great strides in every area of life, including coordination and movement, hand and finger skills, language, and cognitive development.

The most obvious change will be growth. Although the range of "normal" growth varies from one preschooler to the next, your child is likely to grow about 2½ inches taller and gain four to five pounds each year.

Heights and weights will differ depending on family history, your child's sex, nutrition, sleep, and health. Your preschooler's doctor will track your child's weight and height using BMI and height-for-age charts.

The time just after toddlerhood is a whirlwind of activity, filled with fantasy and rich in imagination. However, children in this age group can tend to be bossy, willful, and belligerent. Your job will be to curb out-of-bounds behavior, support growth, and continue to instill healthy lifestyle habits.

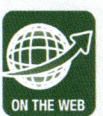

To see a list of milestones for each age, visit:

http://www.choosemyplate.gov/preschoolers/healthy-habits/Milestones.pdf

Growth is one of the best indicators of good health and nutrition in children.

To check your child's BMI and height-for-age charts, visit:

http://www.choosemyplate.gov/preschoolers/growth-input-chart.html

58. Should I be adding foods to my child's diet to compensate for all the running around?

By the time your child is a preschooler, he or she will be eating all the same foods as you. Feed your preschooler a variety of foods to help him or her get the proper amounts of nutrients from all the food groups: grains, vegetables, fruit, dairy, and protein.

Sound nutrition is essential to good health. The American Academy of Pediatrics encourages parents to think of their nutritional choices as health decisions.[10]

One way to achieve that goal is to create a daily food plan. Use it as a general guide to help you feed your child. It will show you what foods and how much of them to offer your child to meet his or her nutritional needs. Don't be concerned if your preschooler doesn't eat everything you put on his or her plate every day. Each child's needs vary, and appetites can change from day to day. The key is to focus on average amounts over time. Food plans are based on average needs by age and activity level. Your preschooler's food needs also depend on how fast he or she is growing and other factors.

Grain products include any food made from wheat, rice, oats, cornmeal, barley, or other cereal grain. Bread, pasta, oatmeal, breakfast cereals, tortillas, and grits are examples of grain products.

Make half of the grains you serve your child whole grains.

They fall into two categories: whole and refined grains. Some products are made from mixtures of these. In general, whole grains offer nutritional advantages and help prevent obesity.

Whole grains are unprocessed and include the entire grain kernel: the bran, germ, and endosperm. Examples are whole-wheat flour, cracked wheat, oatmeal, whole cornmeal, and brown rice. Refined grain products have been milled, a process that removes the bran and germ. This gives the products a finer texture and improves their shelf life, but it also takes out dietary fiber, iron, and many B vitamins. Some examples of refined-grain products are white flour, de-germed cornmeal, white bread, noodles, pretzels, and white rice.

Most refined grains are enriched; certain B vitamins (thiamin, riboflavin, niacin, and folic acid) and iron are added back after processing. Fiber is not put back into enriched grains. If you serve your child refined-grain foods, check the ingredient list to make sure that the word "enriched" is included in the grain name.

Whole grains are defined as the whole unprocessed grains of cereals, such as wheat and maize.

Some grain foods contain significant amounts of bran, which provides fiber, slows digestion (and the return of hunger), and is important for health. However, products with added bran or bran alone, such as oat bran, are not necessarily whole grains.

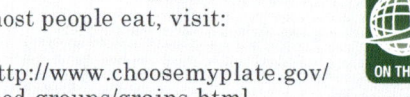
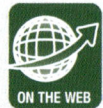

To see a list of grain foods that most people eat, visit:

http://www.choosemyplate.gov/food-groups/grains.html

Check the ingredient list for the words "whole grain" or "whole wheat" to find out if a food is made from a whole grain. Choose whole grains that are higher in dietary fiber. Many preschoolers don't eat enough fiber, and whole-grain foods are an easy way to get fiber into your child's diet.

60. How do vegetables help prevent obesity?

Vegetables are low in calories, high in water content, and help fill your child's stomach; this can prevent overeating or sneaking extra food. They also have many vitamins and minerals that help your preschooler grow and stay healthy. A lot of children dislike or refuse some vegetables, but you can help yours to eat and enjoy a variety of them.

They come in a rainbow of colors. Encourage your child to try them and eat them yourself. Many types are available to choose from, including dark green, red, or orange vegetables. Include them in meals and in snacks. Vegetables come in many forms: fresh, frozen, canned, or dried.

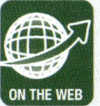 To see a list of many kinds of vegetables you and your child can eat, visit:

http://www.choosemyplate.gov/food-groups/vegetables.html

Vegetables lend themselves to diversity in how they look and taste. They can be prepared and served in many different ways, including whole, cut-up, or pureed. If your preschooler doesn't like one approach, try another. Sprinkle a little no-calorie sweetener on vegetables to make them more

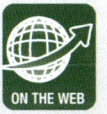 To see a list of tips that can help you and your preschooler eat enough vegetables, visit:

http://www.choosemyplate.gov/food-groups/vegetables-tips.html

appealing or include them in dishes like chili. Vegetables are easy to experiment with. If you use canned vegetables, check the labels and choose ones that say "reduced sodium" or "no salt added."

The amount of vegetables your child needs to eat each day or week depends on his or her age, sex, and level of physical activity. To put potential mealtime battles into perspective, use general guidelines on how much is enough for your preschooler.

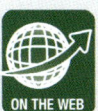 To see charts of recommended total daily vegetable servings and weekly amounts from each type of vegetable, visit:

http://www.choosemyplate.gov/printpages/MyPlateFoodGroups/Vegetables/food-groups.vegetables-amount.pdf

61. Can preschoolers eat as much fruit as they want without putting on extra weight?

Fruits are delicious and provide vital nutrients for fast-growing preschoolers. They're naturally low in fat and calories and rich in vitamin C, which is important for the growth and repair of all body tissues. Nutrition from fruits helps heal cuts and wounds and keep teeth and gums healthy.

Whole fruits (but not fruit juices) contain fiber that can help kids feel full with fewer calories. Nonetheless, parents need to limit

Fill half your child's plate with fruits and vegetables.

how much fruit their preschooler eats each day. No matter how active he or she is, too much of any food, even healthy ones, can put on unwanted weight.

62. Is seafood as good a protein as meat?

With a couple of caveats (see Section 64), seafood is a great choice. It's part of the protein food group, which also includes

To see a list of protein foods and selection tips, visit:

http://www.choosemyplate
.gov/food-groups/protein-foods.html

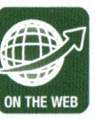

all foods made from meat, poultry, beans and peas, eggs, processed soy products, nuts, and seeds. Beans and peas are also part of the vegetable group. To improve your child's nutrient intake, provide a variety of protein choices.

The health benefits of protein for children are many:

- Meat, poultry, fish, dry beans and peas, eggs, nuts, and seeds supply protein, B vitamins (niacin, thiamin, riboflavin, and B6), vitamin E, zinc, and magnesium.
- Proteins serve as building blocks for bones, muscles, cartilage, skin, and blood. They serve the same function for enzymes, hormones, and vitamins.
- B vitamins help the body release energy, play a vital role in the function of the nervous system, aid in the formation of red blood cells, and help build tissues.
- Iron in proteins carries oxygen in the blood.
- Magnesium builds bones and releases energy from muscles.
- Zinc is needed for biochemical reactions and helps the immune system function properly.

63. What are the negatives associated with protein?

Some proteins are high in saturated fat, which can promote the accumulation of LDL cholesterol (low-density lipoprotein) in your child's arteries. To reduce the risk of future coronary artery disease, even preschoolers need to be careful about eating too much saturated fat.

Proteins that are high in saturated fats include fatty cuts of beef, pork, and lamb; regular (75 to 85% lean) ground beef, sausages, hot dogs, and bacon; some regular luncheon meats, such as bologna and salami; and some poultry, such as duck. Servings of these foods should be limited.

Other protein foods to be careful with are peanuts, walnuts, almonds, and pistachios. It's easy to eat too much of them, but they're high in calories and need to be taken in small portions. They should also be used to replace other proteins, like meat or poultry, rather than being added to what's already on your child's plate. Also, if you let your child eat nuts and seeds, make sure they're unsalted.

64. Can seafood cause mercury poisoning in preschoolers?

The health benefits from eating seafood outweigh the risk of ingesting mercury, which is found in varying levels in different kinds of seafood. Commonly eaten seafood choices in the United States that are lower in mercury include salmon, anchovies, herring, sardines, Pacific oysters, trout, and Atlantic and Pacific mackerel (not king mackerel, which is high in mercury).

65. Why is too much salt bad for little kids?

Nearly all of us eat too much sodium, which is found in salt. This includes most children. The majority of salt comes from processed food and other foods eaten away from the home. The taste for salt is learned. Adding less or no salt and choosing foods lower in salt can help your preschooler learn to like foods with a less salty taste.

Eating less salt is an important way to help preschoolers stay healthy as they grow. It may reduce the risk for high blood pressure and some chronic diseases when they reach adulthood. The recommended daily limit for sodium is less than 1500 milligrams for children one to three years old and less than 1900 milligrams for children four to eight years old.

To eat less salt:

- Use the Nutrition Facts label to compare sodium content for similar foods and to select brands lower in sodium; for example, a cup of tomato soup may have from 700–1260 milligrams of sodium
- Look for "no salt added" or "low sodium" food products
- Prepare foods with little or no added salt
- Before eating canned foods, such as beans, rinse them with water to reduce the amount of salt

Also, look for foods that are good sources of potassium. It counteracts some of sodium's effects on blood pressure. Vegetables like sweet potatoes, beet greens, white beans, potatoes, tomato puree and paste, and soybeans are good foods to choose for potassium, as are fruits like bananas, dried plums (prunes), cantaloupe, and honeydew.

For tips on how to make smart protein choices, visit:

http://www.choosemyplate.gov/ food-groups/protein-foods-tips .html

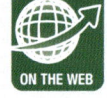

ON THE WEB

66. Do I need to cut back on other dairy foods if my child drinks milk?

The amount of milk and other dairy foods that your preschooler needs to eat depends on age. Recommended daily amounts are shown in the table below.

Daily recommended amounts of dairy to offer girls and boys

DAILY RECOMMENDATION		
Children	2–3 years old	2 cups
	4–8 years old	2½ cups
Girls	9–13 years old	3 cups
	14–18 years old	3 cups
Boys	9–13 years old	3 cups
	14–18 years old	3 cups

To find out what counts as a cup in the dairy food group, visit:

http://www.choosemyplate .gov/food-groups/dairy-counts.html

ON THE WEB

Consuming dairy products provides health benefits, especially improved bone health. Foods from this group provide nutrients that are vital for the health and maintenance of your child's body, including calcium and vitamin D.

Calcium builds bones and teeth and maintains bone mass. Dairy products are the primary source of calcium in American diets. Vitamin D also helps to build and maintain bones. Milk and soy-milk that are fortified with vitamin D are good sources of this nutrient. Other good sources include yogurt and ready-to-eat breakfast cereals fortified with vitamin D.

 Low-fat (1%) or fat-free milk products have little or no solid fat.

67. Can empty calories make a child obese?

Calories from solid fats and added sugars in foods and beverages are empty calories. They add to total calories but provide no vitamins or minerals. Preschoolers can have some empty calories, but too many can fill them up without supplying the nutrients they need. Empty calories can also add more total calories than children need, leading to overweight or obesity.

Some examples of empty calories are sugars or sweeteners in soft drinks, fruit punch, candies, cakes, cookies, pies, and ice cream as well as solid fats in cookies, cakes, pizza, cheese, sausages, fatty meats, butter, and stick margarine.

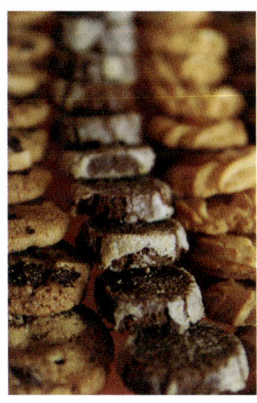

◀ **FIGURE 6.1**
Cookies and sweets © Quinn Dombrowski

Certain foods such as milk, yogurt, and cereals provide important nutrients, but they can also contain some empty calories.

Choose low-fat (1%) or fat-free milk, yogurt, cheese, and cereals that are unsweetened or have no added sugars. These foods have fewer calories but provide the same nutrients as those with more fat or sugar.

To learn more about empty calories, visit:

http://www.choosemyplate.gov/weight-management-calories/calories/empty-calories.html

For example, sweetened yogurt and sweetened breakfast cereals have added sugars. Whole milk and cheese contain solid fat.

Now and then, your child can eat foods that have added sugars or solid fats. However, most daily choices for preschoolers should stay away from empty calories.

Here are some ideas to help you cut down the amount of empty calories your preschooler eats:

INSTEAD OF...	CHOOSE
Regular cheese	Low-fat cheese
Sweetened yogurt	Plain yogurt plus fruit
Whole milk	Fat-free or low-fat milk
Sweetened breakfast cereals	Cereals with little or no added sugar
Cookies	Graham crackers
Fried chicken or fried fish	Baked chicken or fish
French fries	Oven-baked fries
Ice cream or frozen yogurt	Frozen fruits or frozen 100% fruit bars
Soft drinks or fruit punch	Water
Potato chips	Baked chips or whole-grain crackers
Butter or margarine	*Trans*-fat-free tub margarine
Jam or jelly	100% Fruit spread

SOURCE: From the United States Department of Agriculture ChooseMyPlate.gov Daily Food Plan for Preschoolers: Empty Calories. http://www.choosemyplate.gov/preschoolers/daily-food-plans/about-empty-calories.html

To find ideas for meal and snacks for your preschooler, visit:

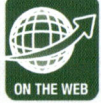

http://www.choosemyplate.gov/preschoolers/meal-and-snack-patterns-ideas.html

68. Should I give my preschooler more snacks than my toddler gets?

Preschoolers should be given two healthy snacks per day. Like toddlers, these should be eaten at a planned time, while seated, and with adult supervision.

69. When can I switch to beverages other than milk or water, like no-calorie sodas and sports drinks?

Continue to offer your preschooler the same beverages as your toddler: low- or fat-free milk, water, and 100% fruit juices in limited quantities.

Water

- When your preschooler is thirsty, water is a good beverage choice. It provides the fluid your child's body needs.
- Be sure to have water on hand when your child is playing outdoors or doing other kinds of physical activities.
- Find out if your preschooler is drinking fluoridated water; it helps build and maintain strong teeth. In many communities, the tap water has fluoride in it. Check with your water supplier to make sure. If your water supply is not fluoridated or is from a well, ask your doctor about a possible need for fluoride supplements.
- Bottled water is not better or safer than regular tap water and is an added expense.
- Flavored or vitamin waters may have added sweeteners. Be sure to read the Nutrition Facts label on these drinks.

Milk

- Milk and milk products provide many vital nutrients that your preschooler needs for growth. Milk is a good choice to offer during meals and snacks.
- While some children don't drink enough milk, others sometimes prefer to fill up on it and avoid other important foods. Preschoolers need about 2–2½ cups of dairy foods each day. Help your child get enough but not too much milk.
- Make sure you serve only pasteurized (not raw) milk to your preschooler.

100% Fruit Juice

- Fresh, frozen, canned and dried fruits provide more fiber than juice. Offer these most often.
- Sweetened beverages, such as fruit punch and fruit drinks, look like fruit juice but they may have little or no fruit in them. These drinks, as well as some flavored

waters, sweetened teas, and sports drinks, provide calories but little or no nutrients.
- Make sure you serve only pasteurized 100% fruit juices to your preschooler.

70. Are preschoolers as picky as toddlers about eating certain foods or new foods?

Yes, they can be just as picky as toddlers. Many preschoolers would rather explore food than eat it. During the preschool years, common behaviors include: unwillingness to try new foods (especially fruits and vegetables), eating only a certain type of food for a period of time, and refusing to eat foods that are red or green, have seeds, or are squishy.

For tips on how to help your child try new foods, visit:

http://www.choosemyplate.gov/preschoolers/picky-eaters/new-foods.html

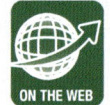
ON THE WEB

Don't try to force your preschooler to eat. Each child's appetite can vary from day to day. Try to balance the amounts eaten over a few days or a week. In most cases, picky behaviors go away on their own.

71. Does my preschooler need as much sleep as my toddler?

Preschoolers (three to five years old) typically sleep 11–13 hours each night, and most do not nap after five years of age. As with toddlers, difficulty falling asleep and waking up during the night are common. As your child's imagination develops, nighttime fears and nightmares become common. In addition, sleepwalking and sleep terrors peak during preschool years.

Some tips for making sure your preschooler gets enough sleep:
- Maintain a regular and consistent sleep schedule
- Have a relaxing bedtime routine that ends in the room where your child sleeps
- Preschoolers should sleep in the same sleeping environment every night, in a room that is cool, quiet, dark, and without a TV [11]

72. How much physical activity does my preschooler need?

Preschoolers love to move. Encourage them to play several times each day. Their activity may happen in short bursts rather than all at once, and it no longer needs to always be led by an adult.

> **FIGURE 6.2**
Preschooler playing

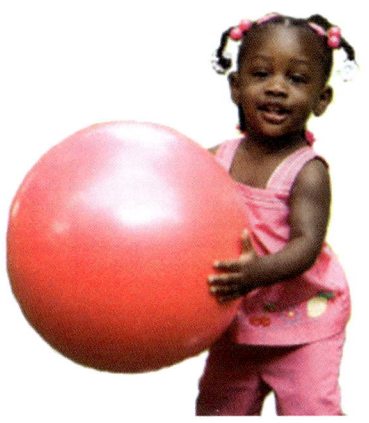

SOURCE: Centers for Disease Control and Prevention

If you wonder if your preschooler is getting enough physical activity, ask yourself the following questions. They can serve as a guide:

- Does he or she play outside several times a day or in a room big enough to run around freely?
- Does your preschooler watch less than two hours of TV daily (including all screen time)?
- Do you make sure that your child doesn't sit for more than 60 minutes at one time?
- Does your preschooler breathe quickly and/or sweat when actively playing?

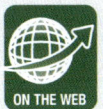

For more information on how much and what kinds of physical activity your preschooler needs, visit:

If you can usually answer yes to these questions, your child is probably getting enough physical activity. The recommended amount is 60 minutes a day.

http://www.cdc.gov/physicalactivity/everyone/guidelines/children.html

73. How can I help my preschooler learn about healthy living in ways that will last?

Every day offers many ways to play, teach, and reinforce the lessons of healthy living—from growing vegetables to learning yoga poses.

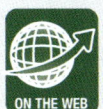

To see how one preschool teacher uses her time with children to help them learn and retain ways to be physically fit and eat wisely, see Video 6.1: Making Health Easier: Healthy Habits in Childcare.

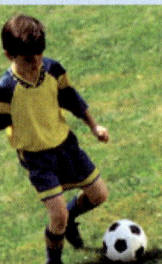

CHAPTER 7

Preventing Obesity in Middle Childhood

74. How will my child change during middle childhood?

Growth will be slow and steady until puberty, which occurs in late middle childhood or early adolescence. However, you'll see rapid cognitive, emotional, and social development.

It's common to see spurts of growth accompanied by increased appetite and food intake. During periods of slower growth, appetite and food intake decrease. Your child's energy requirements will be influenced by growth, physical activity level, and body composition.

Children in middle childhood gain an average of 7 pounds in weight and 2.5 inches in height per year.

Girls tend to have small growth spurts at ages 4.5, 6.5, 8.5, and 10 years, and boys have them slightly later at 4.5, 7, 9, and 10.5 years.

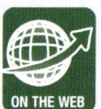

To learn more about physical development during middle childhood, visit:

http://sevencounties.org/poc/view_doc .php?type=doc&id=37674&cn=1272

▶ **FIGURE 7.1**
Friends playing together

75. What developmental milestones should I look for in my 5- to 6-year-old child?

Starting school is a major milestone for the 5- or 6-year-old child. School brings new opportunities, challenges, and rules. Activities require increased impulse control, the ability to obey instructions, get along with others, and avoid disruptive behavior.[12] Progress in school is an important factor in your child's development at this age.

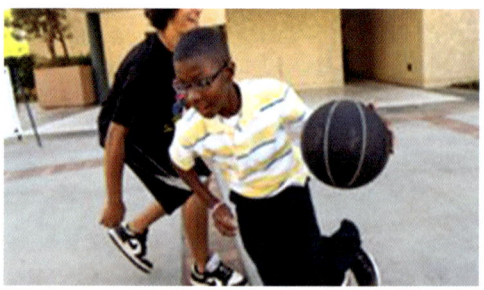

SOURCE: Centers for Disease Control and Prevention

School brings your child into regular contact with the larger world. Cognitive skills will continue to develop along with the ability to understand and communicate in more mature ways. Children want to be liked and accepted by friends and will spend increasing amounts of time with them.

As they learn how their bodies work, children gain the confidence and skills they need to enjoy physical activities or to participate in individual or sport teams. By the age of six, most children will be riding bicycles, using in-line skates or skateboards, and learning to swim.

A sense of body image begins to develop around age six.

Developmental milestones at five years old

Dresses without help

Knows address and telephone number

Can count on fingers

Copies a triangle or square

Draws a person with a head, a body, arms, and legs

Recognizes many letters of the alphabet

Prints some letters

Plays make-believe and dress-up

May be able to skip

76. What changes can I expect to see in my 7- to 8-year-old child?

Seven- or eight-year-old children start to look outside the family for new ideas and activities. They'll take part in school and social activities and spend more time away from home. As their peer group becomes increasingly important, children will identify with kids of the same gender who have similar interests and abilities. They may have a best friend, a milestone in interpersonal development.[12]

School performance remains a barometer of development in all areas (physical, social, affective, and cognitive) of a child's life.

Your seven- to eight-year-old child can start to take on new family responsibilities,

To learn more about the domains of development, visit:

http://www.education.com/reference/article/developmental-milestones-middle-childhood/

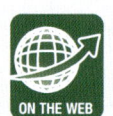

such as making his or her bed, setting the table, and helping with meals. These are the years when your child is forming lifelong habits, including those related to nutrition and physical activity. Continue to serve as a role model and seek opportunities to foster your child's sense of responsibility for choosing positive health behaviors.

77. What changes can I expect to see in my 9- to 10-year-old child?

During middle childhood, muscle strength, motor skills, and stamina increase. Children become coordinated enough to perform complex movements that enable them to participate in a variety of physical activities.

To find out more about health and academics, visit:

http://www.cdc.gov/healthyyouth/health_and_academics/index.htm

By the time they are nine or ten, they have a peer group, are involved in sports, take part in social and community activities, compete at video games, and listen to their favorite music. Friends are of great importance; growing independence from the family is more apparent.

➤ **FIGURE 7.2**
Team sports can play an important role in a school-age child's life

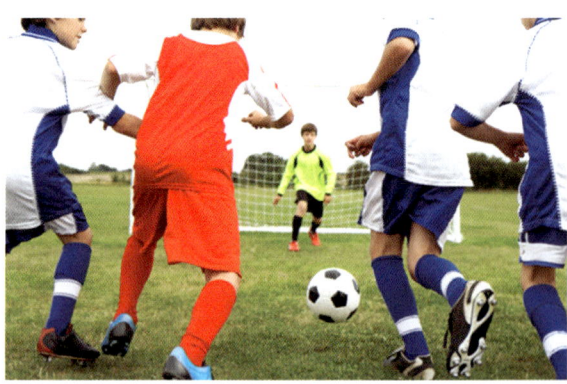

SOURCE: Shutterstock

78. Are there differences in height and weight in prepubescent boys and girls?

Before puberty, there are no significant differences between boys and girls in height, weight, strength, endurance, and motor skill development. They can participate in physical activities as equals.

79. Will my child's weight increase at some point?

Body composition and shape remain relatively constant in middle childhood. However, during preadolescence and early adolescence (9–11 years in girls and 10–12 years in boys) the percentage of body fat increases in preparation for the growth spurt that occurs during adolescence.

Girls gain body fat earlier than boys, and the amount of body fat increase is greater in girls. Preadolescents, especially girls, may look "chunky," but this is part of normal growth and development.

Boys have more muscle, and girls have slightly more body fat. After age eight, girls begin accumulating fat at a faster rate.

80. Are there any body image problems about which I should be aware?

Children may become overly concerned about their physical appearance. Girls may think they're too heavy and start to eat less food or diet. Parents need to reassure them that more body fat at their age is normal and will probably go away. Boys may worry about their stature, muscle size, and strength. They also need to be reassured that their

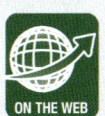

To learn how to promote a positive body image in your child, visit:

http://www.aboutkidshealth.ca/En/ HealthAZ/FamilyandPeerRelations/ AttachmentandEmotions/Pages/ body-image-promoting.aspx

growth is normal and that they'll become bigger and stronger as they get older.

81. Does the risk of eating disorders increase in girls when they reach puberty?

Girls have an increase in body fat at the onset of puberty. Girls, parents, and teachers need to understand this, and girls need to accept the physical changes of puberty; attempts by your child to prevent them can lead to dieting or eating disorders.[12] Crash diets deprive children of essential nutrients during a period of rapid growth and can make matters worse.

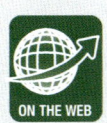

To learn how to talk to you daughter about changes in her body, visit:

http://my.clevelandclinic.org/ childrens-hospital/health-info/ages- stages/adolescence/hic-how-to-talk- to-your-adolescent-girl-about-her- body.aspx

82. Can puberty affect a girl's level of physical activity?

More body fat and a decrease in muscle flexibility during the growth spurt leading up to puberty can increase the risk for overuse injuries. Body changes related to puberty may also cause setbacks in the performance of various sports, putting girls at particularly high risk for becoming more sedentary. At this time, it's important to encourage girls to continue their physical activities and for you to serve as an active role model.

To find out more about precautions for the young female athlete, visit: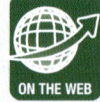

http://my.clevelandclinic.org/childrens-hospital/health-info/ages-stages/childhood/hic-Precautions-for-the-Young-Female-Athlete.aspx

83. Do I need to feed my daughter less as she adds fat during puberty?

To find out more about food and physical activity recommendations for children between 6–11 years of age, visit: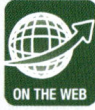

http://www.cnpp.usda.gov/mypyramid-forkids.htm

Your daughter should continue to eat recommended portions of healthy and nutritious foods.

84. What should I do if my child has problems adjusting to eating at school?

To learn more about access to healthy drinking water at schools, visit: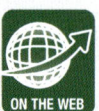

http://www.cdc.gov/healthyyouth/npao/wateraccess.htm

Praise your child for making healthy food choices and encourage him or her to continue doing so. Schools are in a unique position to promote healthy eating and help ensure appropriate food and nutrient intake among students. They provide opportunities to eat an array of foods and beverages throughout the school day and enable students to learn about and practice healthy eating behaviors. For example, as a healthy alternative to sugar-sweetened beverages, they can provide access to safe, free drinking water.

For information on teaching kids about nutrition, visit: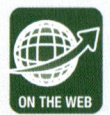

http://www.schoolnutrition.org/Content.aspx?id=94

85. What should I expect my child's school to do when it comes to helping him or her make healthy food choices?

Schools should make sure that only nutritious and appealing

foods and beverages are offered in cafeterias, vending machines, snack bars, and school stores. In addition, nutrition education should be part of a comprehensive health education curriculum.

86. My child is having orthodontia. Does this make a difference in what he or she can eat?

If children are missing teeth, growing permanent teeth, or having orthodontic treatment, they may have difficulty chewing certain foods, such as raw vegetables or meat. They may need foods that are easier to eat, such as chopped hamburger or low-fat or fat-free cottage cheese.

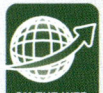 To learn more about orthodontia in kids, visit:

http://kidshealth.org/ teen/your_body/medical_care/ braces.html

87. What nutrients do I need to pay special attention to during middle childhood?

Children need a variety of nutritious foods that give them sufficient calories, protein, carbohydrates, fat, vitamins, and minerals. Breakfast is one of the more important sources of nutrients for children.

 Eating a healthy breakfast can promote success in school. It's associated with improved cognitive function (especially memory), reduced absenteeism, and improved mood.[13]

Calcium intake is also of special concern during middle childhood. Few school-aged children get enough of it, but having adequate amounts is essential for strong bones and teeth. Children who drink large amounts of juice, soft drinks, or sports drinks are at risk for inadequate calcium intake. Children two to eight years old need to drink two cups of low-fat (1%) or fat-free (skim) milk per day or consume the equivalent from other milk products (cheese, yogurt). Those aged nine and older need to drink three cups of low-fat (1%) or fat-free (skim) milk or eat the equivalent from cheese, yogurt, or other dairy products. One 8-ounce glass of milk contains about 300 mg of calcium.

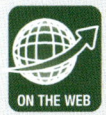 To learn about ten signs of nutritional deficiencies in children, visit:

http://www.weedemandreap.com/10-signs-of-nutritional-deficiencies-in-children/

Vitamin D is also a nutrient to keep an eye on. Children who don't get 400 IU per day of vitamin D through fortified milk (100 IU per 8 ounces) or fortified foods, such as cereals or should take a vitamin D supplement of 400 IU per day.

88. What kinds of physical activities should my child do?

Encourage your child to participate for an hour a day in physical activities that are age-appropriate, enjoyable, and offer variety. Make sure your child does three types of activities at least three days per week: aerobics, such as running or bicycling; muscle strengthening, such as climbing trees or sit-ups; and bone strengthening, such as jumping rope or playing basketball. Physical activities that can be sustained throughout life are ideal (for example, walking, hiking, biking, skating, dancing, and swimming).

Age-appropriate physical activities

AGE	MOTOR SKILLS BEING DEVELOPED	APPROPRIATE PHYSICAL ACTIVITIES
5–6 years	Fundamental (for example, running, galloping, jumping, hopping, skipping, throwing, catching, striking, or kicking)	• Activities that focus on having fun and developing motor skills rather than on competition • Simple activities that require little instruction • Repetitive activities that don't require complex motor and cognitive skills (for example, running, swimming, tumbling, or throwing or catching a ball)
7–9 years	Fundamental Transitional (for example, throwing for distance or accuracy)	• Activities that focus on having fun and developing motor skills rather than on competition • Activities with flexible rules • Activities that require little instruction • Activities that do not require complex motor and cognitive skills (for example, entry-level baseball or soccer)

AGE	MOTOR SKILLS BEING DEVELOPED	APPROPRIATE PHYSICAL ACTIVITIES
10–11 years	Transitional Complex (such as playing basketball)	• Activities that continue to focus on having fun and developing motor skills rather than on competition • Activities that require entry-level complex motor and cognitive skills • Activities that continue to emphasize motor skill development but begin to incorporate instruction on strategy and teamwork

SOURCE: Hagan, J.F., et al. (2008). *Bright Futures: Guidelines for Health Supervision of Infants, Children, and Adolescents*, 3rd ed.[1]

89. My child likes to watch TV, play computer games, and has no interest in sports. How can I help make physical activity a regular part of his or her life?

Sedentary habits in school-aged children are linked to increased risk of obesity and heart disease in adults. You can have a major impact on your child's level of physical activity during middle childhood. Limit screen time (including computers, tablets, and cell phones) to one or two hours a day, and designate a specific time for physical activity that he or she enjoys. Be sure to give positive feedback to your child when he or she is physically active.

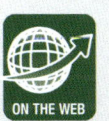

To find out how to put limits on screen time, visit:

http://www.mayoclinic.org/healthy-living/childrens-health/in-depth/children-and-tv/art-20047952?pg=1

Make opportunities for being active readily available, such as swimming or dancing lessons, playing outside, and walking. Participate with your child in physical activity: take a walk together, shoot some hoops, throw a ball back and forth, or teach your child how to play baseball. Your influence will show that physical activity can be fun and have a lasting positive effect. Children can also be influenced to get and stay active by other family members, peers, coaches, and teachers.

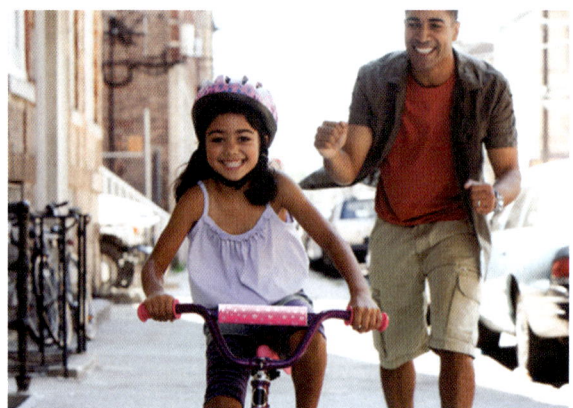

◄ FIGURE 7.3
Child riding a bicycle

To learn more about how to motivate your child to be active, visit:

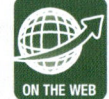
ON THE WEB

http://kidshealth.org/parent/nutrition_center/staying_fit/schoolage_active.html?tracking=P_RelatedArticle

Fun, a feeling of competence, and a variety of options encourage physical activity. Feelings of failure, boredom, and embarrassment can be reasons to become sedentary. Competition and rigid rules also discourage participation in sports.

90. My child plays a lot of sports. Is it still necessary for him or her to take physical education in school?

Many schools have eliminated physical education due to budget cuts or to divert resources into test preparation. If your child's school offers physical education, he or she should take advantage of it. Physical education can help your child learn about the importance of daily activity, develop motor skills, keep physically fit, and introduce him or her to a variety of ways to stay active. Some of these might become lifelong pursuits.

See Video 7.1: Children and Adolescents: The Physical and Activity Guidelines in Action,

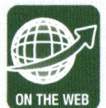
ON THE WEB

91. My neighborhood isn't safe for outdoor play. How can my child still be physically active?

As a parent, you play a key role in promoting school and community changes that make it easier to be physically active. Encourage your child's school to offer after-hours and weekend physical activity programs. Help your child get involved with community organizations, Boys and Girls Clubs, recreation centers, churches or other religious venues that provide opportunities for physical activity. Work with community leaders to seek federal and/or state funding to build safe places to play and be active (for example, walking and biking paths, playgrounds, parks, basketball and tennis courts, and baseball diamonds).

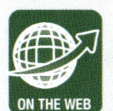 To find out how communities across America are making it easier to be physically active, visit:

http://www.cdc.gov/nccdphp/dch/programs/CommunitiesPutting-PreventiontoWork/action/physical_activity.htm

92. Does indoor play work as well as outdoor activity?

Soft equipment can make indoor play a viable option. Your child can do modified versions of bowling, basketball, darts, and golf. Other options include dancing, stretching, and doing calisthenics and aerobic activity.

93. Does my child still need as much sleep as when he or she was younger?

Well-rested children are better able to focus attention and learn during classes or extracurricular activities. They're more likely to be in a better mood than poorly rested peers and follow rules at home and school. They're also less likely to become obese.[14]

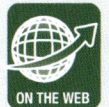 To find out more about sleep and your school-aged child, see:

http://www.nationwidechildrens.org/sleep-in-school-aged-children

Children in middle childhood need about 10–11 hours of sleep each night. By this age, most of them will be able to get all of their necessary sleep in a single overnight session, enabling them to attend school and other after-school activities without the need for a nap. For children six to ten years of age, the suggested bedtime is 8:00–9:00 p.m.

Preventing Obesity in Adolescence

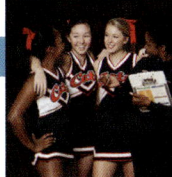

94. What will adolescence be like?

Adolescence is the transition between childhood and adulthood. One of the most dynamic periods of human development,

To learn more about how your adolescent might feel about various aspects of life, see:

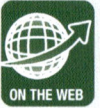

http://www.youtube.com/watch?v=f5
MYXo8amUs

it is characterized by dramatic physical, cognitive, social, and emotional changes.[15] These years hold a number of challenges for you and your child as he or she seeks growing independence, searches for his or her identity, and gets increasingly concerned with appearance and peer acceptance. Decisions made during adolescence can have immediate and lifelong effects.

95. How fast will my adolescent grow?

The rate of growth during adolescence is second only to that which takes place during your child's first year of life. During this period, teens complete the last 15–20% of their adult height, gain 50% of their adult body weight, and accumulate up to 40% of their adult skeletal mass.[15]

96. What other changes can I expect to see?

Females have a normal accumulation of fat in the hips, thighs, and buttocks. Fat accumulation ranges from 15–18% of body weight before puberty to 20–25% at its end. Males have a slight weight gain before a growth spurt between the ages of 9–13, a decrease in body fat during the growth spurt, and an increase after puberty (about 15–18% of body weight by the age of 18). Some males will mature later than their peers. They need reassurance from parents and their doctor that their growth is normal.[16]

To find out more about your adolescent's physical development, visit:

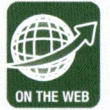

http://www.nlm.nih.gov/medlineplus/ency/
article/002003.htm

97. When does adolescence start and end?

According to the American Academy of Pediatrics,[16] adolescence runs from ages 11–21. However, it's not just one long stretch of trying times for parents. The Academy divides the years into three stages: early adolescence (ages 11–14), middle adolescence (ages 15–17), and late adolescence (ages 18–21).

The first stage is characterized by the changes of puberty and a growing capacity for abstract thought, although it is oriented toward the present. The second stage is one of independence, experimentation, future-oriented thinking, and greater problem-solving abilities. The third and last stage is a time of important personal, educational, and vocational decisions. Those in late adolescence have refined abilities to reason logically and solve problems.[16]

The physical, cognitive, and emotional development stages of adolescence are shown in the table below.

STAGES OF ADOLES-CENCE	PHYSICAL DEVELOPMENT	CONGNITIVE DEVELOP-MENT	SOCIAL-EMOTIONAL DEVELOPMENT
Early Adolescence **Approxi-mately 11–13 years of age**	• Puberty: grow body hair, increase perspiration and oil production in hair and skin, Girls – breast and hip development, onset of menstruation Boys – growth in testicles and penis, wet dreams, deepening of voice. • Tremendous phyical growth: gain height and weight • Greater sexual interest	• Growing capacity for abstract thought • Mostly interested in present with limited thought to the future • Intellectual interests expand and become more important • Deeper moral thinking	• Struggle with sense of identity • Feel awkward about one's self and one's body; worry about being normal • Realize that parents are not perfect: increased conflict with parents • Increased influence of peer group • Desire for indepen-dence • Tendency to return to "childish" behavior, particularly when stressed • Moodiness • Rule- and limit-testing • Greater interest in privacy

Continued

Continued

STAGES OF ADOLES- CENCE	PHYSICAL DEVELOPMENT	CONGNITIVE DEVELOP- MENT	SOCIAL-EMOTIONAL DEVELOPMENT
Middle Adolescence **Approxi- mately 14–18 years of age**	• Puberty is completed • Physical growth slows for girls, continues for boys	• Continued growth of capacity for abstract thought • Greater capacity for setting goals • Interest in moral reasoning • Thinking about the meaning of life	• Intense self-involve- ment, changing between high expectations and poor self-concept • Continued adjustment to changing body, worries about being normal • Tendency to distance selves from parents, continued drive for independence • Driven to make friends and greater reliance on them, popularity can be an important issue • Feelings of love and passion
Late Adolescence **Approxi- mately 19–21 years of age**	• Young women, typically, are fully developed • Young men continue to gain height, weight, muscle mass, and body hair	• Ability to think ideas through • Ability to delay gratification • Examination of inner experiences • Increased concern for future • Continued interest in moral reasoning	• Firmer sense of identity • Increased emotional stability • Increased concern for others • Increased independence and self-reliance • Peer relationships remain important • Development of more serious relationships • Social and cultural traditions regain some of their importance

SOURCE: Adapted from the American Academy of Child and Adolescent's Facts for Families.© All right reserved. 2008

98. What are the developmental milestones of early adolescence?

Puberty is perhaps the key developmental milestone of early adolescence. Hormones change as it begins. Physical effects in boys include growth of the penis and testicles, height increase, change in body shape, erections with ejaculation, growth of facial and body hair, and a deeper voice. Girls have breast development, changes in body shape and height, growth of pubic and body hair, and the start of menstruation.

Your teen might be worried about these changes and how they are viewed by others. Parents should let them know that healthy body weight is based on genetically determined size and shape rather than on a socially defined ideal weight. They should also discourage dieting and emphasize a healthy lifestyle instead.[17]

This will also be a time when your adolescent may face peer pressure to drink alcohol, smoke cigarettes, use drugs, and have sex. Other challenges can include eating disorders, depression, and problems with peers and family.

At this age, teens make more of their own choices about friends, sports, studying, and school. They become more independent, with their own personality and interests, but parents are still very important.

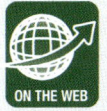
To find out how to help your teen through puberty, watch:

http://www.youtube.com/watch?v=R-MaUtumItw

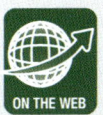
To find out how peer pressure paves the way to adulthood, visit:

http://online.wsj.com/news/articles/SB10001424127887324520904578551462766909232

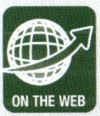
To learn about normal early adolescent development in the middle-school and high-school years, visit:

http://www.aacap.org/AACAP/Families_and_Youth/Facts_for_Families/Facts_for_Families_Pages/Normal_Adolescent_Development_Part_I_57.aspx

99. What are the key changes during middle adolescence?

Older teens (15–17 years old) go through a time of change in how they think, feel, and interact with others. They're also very focused on how their bodies grow. Most girls will be physically mature by now and will have completed puberty. Boys might still be maturing physically.

Your teen could have concerns about body size, shape, or weight. Eating disorders can also be common, especially among girls. These should be assessed by your child's doctor, and treatment should be provided if needed.

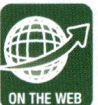

"People spend their childhood learning to be like their parents, and their adolescence learning who they are and how they are different from their parents." — Miriam Kaufman, MD, Department of Pediatrics, University of Toronto, Toronto, Ontario

During this time, your adolescent is developing his or her unique personality and opinions. Relationships with friends are still important, yet teens will have other interests as they develop a clearer sense of who they are. This is an important time to prepare for more independence and responsibility; many teenagers start working, and others will leave home soon after high school.

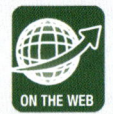

To learn more about your teen's growing independence and how you can play a positive role, visit:

http://raisingchildren.net.au/articles/independence_teenagers.html/context/1158

Cognitive capacities increase dramatically in this phase. Developing an identity and becoming an independent young adult are also central to adolescence.

100. What are the key changes in late adolescence?

Late adolescence marks the final transition from childhood to young adulthood. Generally, physical development is complete, and by this point, adolescents have typically developed a sense of self-identity and a rational and realistic conscience. They've also refined their moral, religious, and sexual values. However, they're still developing cognitively; new research suggests that this process may continue into their 30s.[18]

To learn more about the cognitive development of your teen, visit:

http://sevencounties.org/poc/view_doc.php?type=doc&id=41156&cn=1310

Society regards those in late adolescence as adults. They can legally drive, vote, smoke, drink alcohol, give consent, and enter into contracts. Legal infractions create a permanent criminal record.

After completing high school, young adults join the work force or the military or go to college. Living situations vary widely. They might be on their own, have a roommate or partner, or join a group setting.

101. Will my teen's nutrient needs change with all these physical developments?

Nutrient needs are greatest during peak periods of growth. The mean age of the growth spurt into puberty starts at 9.5 years in females, and 11.5 years in males. About two years after menarche, most physical growth in females is completed. The mean age of a girl's first period is 12.5 years. Males start puberty about two years later, and usually experience their major growth spurts and increase in muscle mass during middle adolescence (15–17 years of age).

102. Will my child's adolescence drive us apart?

Your teen's relationship with you and other adults may start to change during the early stages of adolescence. Some families will suffer with teen mood swings and ongoing arguments over new friends, behaviors, and lifestyles, but most will enjoy an orderly progression to independent decision-making. Only 5–15% of teenagers suffer extreme emotional turmoil, become rebellious, or have major conflicts with their parents.

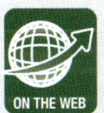 ON THE WEB

To find out more about teenage rebellion, visit:

http://powertochange.com/family/rebellion/

103. How can I ease tension and conflict through the teen years?

Arguments every now and then are common, but authoritative parents (defined as accepting, firm, and democratic) can build a strong protective bond between themselves and their adolescent. The key is a balanced approach that combines unconditional love with clear boundaries (family rules, limits, and expectations) and consistent enforcement of discipline.[16]

 NOTE

Parents tend to influence a young person's long-term decisions, such as career choices, values, and morals. Their friends are more likely to influence short-term choices, such as appearance and interests.

Positive cumulative experiences from childhood to adolescence provide a strong foundation to rely on during what can be tumultuous times. For a young teen, strong self-esteem and self-confidence can help him or her successfully navigate the challenges of adolescence.

You can take certain steps to help him or her:

- Make sure your teen knows about the importance of wearing seatbelts. Motor vehicle crashes are the leading cause of death among 12–14-year-olds.
- Talk about the dangers of drugs, drinking, smoking, and risky sexual activity. Ask what he or she knows and thinks about these issues; share your thoughts and feelings with him or her. Listen to what your teen says and answer questions honestly and directly.
- Meet and get to know his or her friends.
- Show an interest in your teen's school life.
- Help teens make healthy choices while encouraging them to make their own decisions.
- Respect your teen's opinions and take into account his or her thoughts and feelings. It's important that he or she knows that you are listening.
- If there is a conflict, be clear about goals and expectations (like getting good grades, keeping things clean, and showing respect). At the same time, allow your teen to have a say on how to reach those goals (such as when and how to study or clean).

105. How can I help my older teen meet new challenges?

Ways to help older teens meet new challenges of adolescence are to:

- Show interest in school and extracurricular activities and encourage your teen to get involved in such activities as sports, music, theater, and art
- Encourage your teen to volunteer and be involved in civic activities in your community
- Compliment him or her and celebrate his or her efforts and accomplishments

- Be affectionate and spend time together doing things that you both enjoy
- Respect your teen's opinion and listen to him or her without judging or playing down concerns
- If your teen works, use the opportunity to talk about expectations, responsibilities, and other ways of behaving respectfully in a public setting
- Respect his or her need for privacy
- Encourage teens to develop solutions to problems or conflicts, help them make good decisions, create opportunities for them to use their own judgment, and be available for advice and support
- Set clear rules for your teen when he or she is home alone or with friends
- Encourage your adolescent to get enough sleep, exercise, and eat healthy, balanced meals

106. What serious risks does my teen face during adolescence?

During the transition from childhood to adulthood, adolescents establish patterns of behavior and make important lifestyle choices. Serious health and safety issues that confront teens include motor vehicle crashes, violence, dating problems, drunk driving, substance abuse, and risky sexual behaviors.

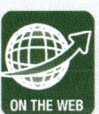

To learn how to protect your teen's sexual health, visit:

http://www.mayoclinic.org/healthy-living/sexual-health/in-depth/teens-and-sex/art-20045927?pg=1

107. What can I do to help my teen stay safe?

Motor vehicle crashes are the leading cause of death from unintentional injury among teens, yet few takes measures to reduce their risk of injury. Steer your teen in the right direction; talk about the dangers of driving and how to be safe on the road.

Unintentional injuries from taking part in sports and other activities are common. Encourage or remind your adolescent to wear a helmet when riding a bike

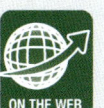

To find out more about what you can do keep your child safe on the road, see Video 8.1: Parents are the Key to Safe Teen Drivers.

or a skateboard or using inline skates, playing contact sports, or while on a motorcycle, snowmobile, or all-terrain vehicle.

Suicide is the third leading cause of death among youths 15–24 years of age. Talk to your teen about his or her concerns and pay attention to any changes in behavior. Ask if he or she has any suicidal thoughts, particularly if he or she seems sad or depressed. Asking about suicidal thoughts will not bring them on; it will just let your adolescent know that you care about how he or she feels. If necessary, seek professional help.

To learn more about teen suicide and how to prevent it, visit:

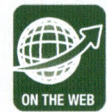

ON THE WEB

http://www.nami.org/Content/Content-Groups/Helpline1/Teenage_Suicide.htm

If your teen uses interactive Internet media such as games, chat rooms, and instant messaging, encourage him or her to make good decisions about what gets posted and the amount of time he or she spends on these activities.

To find out more about how your teen can be safe online, visit:

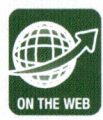

ON THE WEB

http://www.pamf.org/teen/life/risktaking/internet.html

Talk with your adolescent and help him or her plan ahead for difficult or uncomfortable situations. Discuss what to do if he or she is under pressure to have sex or is offered a ride by someone who's been drinking.

To find out what to do if your teen starts hanging around with an undesirable peer group, visit:

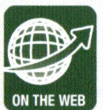

ON THE WEB

http://aspeneducation.crchealth.com/articles/article-peer-groups/

Know where your teen is and whether an adult is present. Make plans for when he or she will call you, where you can find him or her, and what time you expect him or her to be home.

Discuss the importance of choosing friends who do not act in dangerous or unhealthy ways.

108. How will my teen's lifestyle change as he or she enters young adulthood and leaves home?

The transition to young adulthood exposes adolescents to new relationships, lifestyles, dietary patterns, and exercise habits. Responsibilities and life stresses increase, as do access to drugs and alcohol. With their food decisions no longer supervised, personal health behaviors might change. For some young adults, independent living creates opportunities to improve their nutrition and physical activity levels. For others, nutritious foods may be seen as unaffordable or inconvenient. Access to formal exercise programs or team participation may be limited; gym membership may be beyond their financial reach.

109. How can I help my child maintain healthy lifestyle habits?

The dietary and physical activity behaviors of adolescents are influenced by many sectors of society, including communities, schools, medical care providers, faith-based institutions, government agencies, the media, and the food/beverage, fashion, and entertainment industries. The government provides dietary tools and information to cut through the clutter.

Schools play a particularly critical role by establishing a safe and supportive environment with policies and practices that engage adolescents in healthy behaviors. Schools also provide opportunities for students to learn about and practice sound eating and physical activity levels.

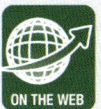

To find out about the Dietary Guidelines for Americans 2010 [19] and related information, visit:

http://www.health.gov/dietaryguidelines/2010.asp#overview

To go directly to the Dietary Guidelines for Americans 2010, visit:

http://www.health.gov/dietaryguidelines/dga2010/DietaryGuidelines2010.pdf

If your adolescent still lives at home, continue to serve a variety of healthful foods and share at least one meal as a family. Eating together will help your teen make better choices about the foods he or she eats, promote normal weight, and give family members time to talk with each other.

In addition, teens who eat meals with their families are more likely to get better grades and less likely to smoke, drink, or use drugs. They're also less likely to get into fights, think about suicide, or engage in sexual activity.

110. How can I help my adolescent stay physically active?

Today's environment offers many opportunities for being sedentary. To overcome this tendency, being physically active must be

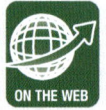

To see a summary of why we need to balance the calories we eat with our level of physical activity, see Video 8.2: Finding Balance.

a lifelong, conscious decision. This is easier to do when being active starts early in life, and adolescents develop skills and pastimes they can enjoy throughout their adulthood.[15]

Some adolescents are aware of diseases that affect their family or community, such as obesity, diabetes, or cardiovascular disease. This knowledge may make them receptive to actions they can take to lower their risk of getting these illnesses. Health care professionals can link exercise with reduced risk of diseases and/or disabilities that affect members of their family, neighbors, and perhaps many other people within their community.[15] This knowledge can often serve as an incentive to remain physically active.

111. Will vigorous activity affect my son's growth and physical development during adolescence?

Encourage your son to eat a variety of healthy foods for growth, physical development, and his level of activity. Growth and physical development in teens who are training and competing in vigorous physical activities, especially those that emphasize low body weight (such as distance running, gymnastics, and basketball), may be compromised if they add excess weight.[15]

112. Can my daughter participate in physical activity during her period?

Yes. In fact, benefits accrue to girls who are physically active during their periods (such as less cramping and lighter menstrual flow). Adolescents who experience symptoms like severe cramping, nausea, vomiting, headache, lightheadedness, and heavy flow tend to avoid physical activity during their periods. These symptoms can usually be managed, but your daughter should still be evaluated by a health professional.

To find out more about exercising during menstruation, visit:

http://www.livestrong.com/article/467253-exercise-during-menstruation/

113. When can my teen lift weights?

Most teens can safely lift weights with proper training and supervision. They should not try to lift maximal amounts until they reach physical maturity (usually 16 years of age for males and 2 years after menarche for females). Adolescents should not try to lift weight beyond their capabilities, and excessive repetitions and power lifting are not recommended.

➤ **FIGURE 8.1**
Teen lifting weights © Ivonne Wierink

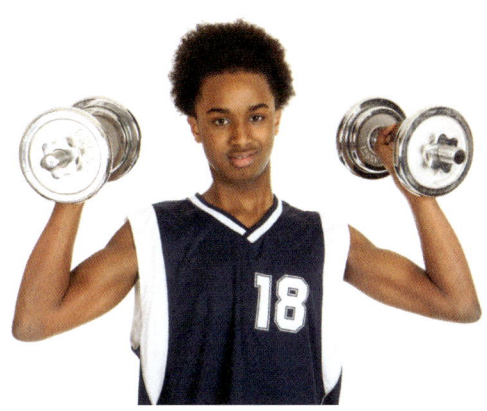

SOURCE: Shutterstock

114. Does fast growth during adolescence increase risk of injury?

Muscle strains, sprains, and overuse injuries are possible during growth spurts. They happen occasionally, but are not a reason to avoid physical activity.

115. Do hours of sleep affect what and how my teen eats?

Teens who sleep less than seven hours per night are more likely to consume fast foods and less likely to eat fruits and vegetables compared to those who sleep more than seven or eight hours a night. All told, adolescents should sleep about nine and one-quarter hours a night. Most of them should go to bed around 11:30 p.m.

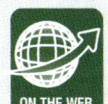
ON THE WEB

To find out more about your teen and sleep, visit:

http://sleepfoundation.org/sleep-topics/teens-and-sleep

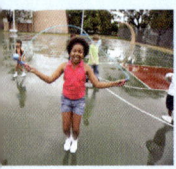

References and Endnotes

CHAPTER 4

1. (2013). *Study finds strong genetic component to childhood obesity*. Available at: http://www.sciencedaily.com/releases/2013/03/130326112234.htm. Accessed April 19, 2014.

2. Eden A.N., Moore B.J., Forman A. (2014). *Fit From the Start: How to Prevent Childhood Obesity in Infancy* (in press). Shape Up America, Clyde Park, MT.

3. American Academy of Pediatricians/healthychildren.org. Infant Food & Feeding Baby 0–12 months. http://www.aap.org/en-us/Pages/Default.aspx. Accessed April 20, 2014.

4. Institute of Medicine. (2011). *Early Childhood Obesity Prevention*. Washington, DC: The National Academies Press.

CHAPTER 5

1. Holt, K. (2011). *Bright Futures: Nutrition, Pocket Guide*, 3rd ed., American Academy of Pediatrics.

2. (2009). *Caring for Your Baby and Young Child: Birth to Age 5*. American Academy of Pediatrics. Atlanta, GA: A&B Media Services.

3. (2011). *Early Childhood Obesity Prevention Policies*. Washington, D.C: Institute of Medicine.

4. Bell, J.F., Zimmerman, F.J. (2010). *Shortened Nighttime Sleep Duration in Early Life and Subsequent Childhood Obesity*. Arch Pediatr Adolesc Med; 164(9): 840–845.

5. Taveras, E.M., Gillman, M.W., Pena, M., Redline, S., Rifas-Shiman, S.L. (2014). *Chronic Sleep Curtailment and Adiposity*. Pediatrics; 133(6): 1013–1022.

CHAPTER 6

1. American Academy of Pediatrics. (2014). healthychildren.org. Available at: http://www.healthychildren.org/English/ages-stages/preschool/Pages/default.aspx. Accessed June 2, 2014.

2. National Sleep Foundation. (2013). *Children and Sleep*. Available at: http://sleepfoundation.org/sleep-topics/children-and-sleep/page/0%2C2/. Accessed June 2, 2014.

CHAPTER 7

1. Hagan, J.F., Shaw, J.S., and Duncan, P., eds. (2008). *Bright Futures Guidelines for Health Supervision of Infants, Children, and Adolescents*, 3rd ed. Elk Grove Village, IL: American Academy of Pediatrics.

2. Hoyland, A., Dye, L., and Lawton, C.L. (2009). *A Systematic Review of the Effect of Breakfast on the Cognitive Performance of Children and Adolescents*. Nutr Res Rev.; 22: 220–243.

3. Nixon, G.M., Thompson, J.M., Han, D.Y., Becroft, D.M., Clark, P.M., Robinson, E., Waldie, K.E., Wild, C.J., Black, P.N., Mitchell, E.A. (2008). *Short Sleep Duration in Middle Childhood: Risk Factors and Consequences*. Sleep; 31: 71–78.

CHAPTER 8

1. Study finds strong genetic component to childhood obesity. 2013; http://www.sciencedaily.com/releases/2013/03/130326112234.htm. Accessed April 19, 2014.

2. Eden AN, Moore BJ, Forman A. *Fit From the Start: How to Prevent Childhood Obesity in Infancy (in press)*. Clyde Park, MT: Shape Up America; 2014.

3. Yager PH, Cummings BM, Whalen MJ, Noviski N. Nighttime telecommunication between remote staff intensivists and bedside personnel in a pediatric intensive care unit: a retrospective study. *Crit. Care Med.* 2012;40(9):2700-2703.

4. Institute of Medicine (IOM). *Early Childhood Obesity Prevention*. Washington, DC: The National Academies Press; 2011.

5. Holt K. *Bright Futures: Nutrition, 3rd Edition Pocket Guide*. Elk Grove Village, IL: American Academy of Pediatrics; 2011.

6. American Academy of Pediatrics. *Caring for Your Baby and Young Child: Birth to Age 5* Atlanta, GA: A&B Media Services; 2009.

7. Institute of Medicine (IOM). *Early Childhood Obesity Prevention Policies*. Washington, D.C.2011.

8. Bell JF, Zimmerman FJ. Shortened nighttime sleep duration in early life and subsequent childhood obesity. *Archives of pediatrics & adolescent medicine*. 2010;164(9):840-845.

9. Taveras EM, Gillman MW, Pena M, Redline S, Rifas-Shiman SL. Chornic sleep curtailment and adiposity. 2014; http://pediatrics. aappublications.org/content/early/2014/05/14/peds.2013-3065. Accessed May 21, 2014.

10. American Academy of Pediatrics. healthychildren.org. 2014; http://www.healthychildren.org/English/ages-stages/preschool/Pages/default.aspx. Accessed June 2, 2014.

11. National Sleep Foundation. Children and Sleep. 2013; http://sleepfoundation.org/sleep-topics/children-and-sleep/page/0%2C2/. Accessed June 2, 2014.

12. Hagan JF, Shaw JS, Duncan P, eds. *Bright Futures Guidelines for Health Supervision of Infants, Children, and Adolescents--Third Edition*. Elk Grove Village, IL: American Academy of Pediatrics; 2008.

13. Hoyland A, Dye L, Lawton CL. A systematic review of the effect of breakfast on the cognitive performance of children and adolescents. *Nutrition research reviews*. 2009;22(2):220-243.

14. Nixon GM, Thompson JM, Han DY, et al. Short sleep duration in middle childhood: risk factors and consequences. *Sleep*. 2008;31(1):71-78.

15. American Academy of Pediatrics. Bright Futures in Practice: Physical Activity. Third:http://www.brightfutures.org/physicalactivity/ad/1.html. Accessed July 8, 2014.

16. American Academy of Pediatrics. Bright Futures Guidelines for Health Supervision of Infants, Children, and Adolescents. http://www.brightfutures.org/bf2/pdf/pdf/MC.pdf. Accessed May 30, 2014.

17. Holt K. *Bright Futures: Nutrition, 3rd Edition Pocket Guide*. American Academy of Pediatrics;2011.

18. Weinberger DR, Elvevag B, Giedd JN. *The Adolescent Brain: Work in Progress. The National Campaign to Prevent Teen Pregnancy*. Washington, D.C.2005.

19. U.S. Department of Agriculture and U.S. Department of Health and Human Services. *Dietary Guidelines for Americans, 2010, 7th Edition*. Washington, D.C.: U.S. Government Printing Office;2010.

PART THREE

ASSESSING AND TREATING OBESITY

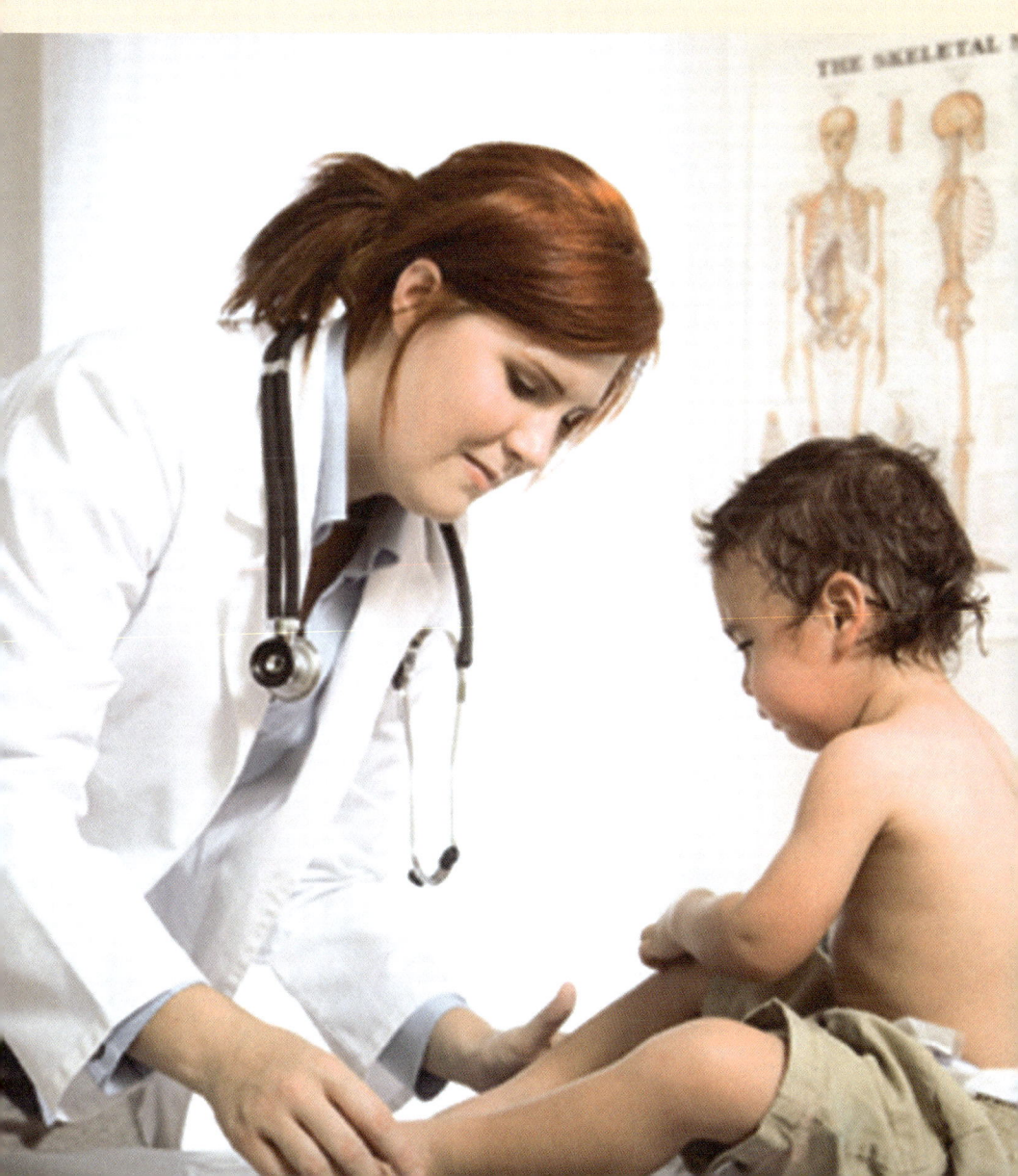

In Part Three, we describe the role of the physician in screening and assessing childhood obesity and its comorbidities. We discuss why it's important to have a skilled and knowledgeable doctor on your side and how he or she can help you do what's best for your child. We also cover various treatment options including lifestyle interventions, medication, and weight loss surgery.

CHAPTER 9

The Role of the Physician in Childhood Obesity

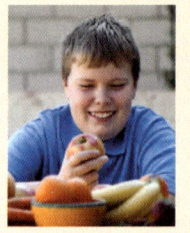

CHAPTER 10

Treatment Options for Childhood Obesity

The Role of the Physician in Childhood Obesity

116. How can I tell if my pediatrician is competent to deal with childhood obesity?

Physicians are key players in the fight against childhood obesity. Even though large numbers of them still feel that they lack the time or expertise to effectively deal with the disease, many others have taken on the challenge. To tell them apart, look for: [1]

- Routine documentation of BMI, and the means to track it consistently and accurately (this includes having reliable and calibrated scales for infants and children, recumbent infant length boards, and wall mounted stadiometers to measure height)

A Stadiometer is an instrument for measuring standing or sitting height.

- An office staff trained to accurately measure weight and height, calculate BMI, and plot measures on growth curves

- Obesity prevention messages, goals, or recommendations to all children through posters, handouts, brochures, and other materials, with reinforcement of messages at every visit

- Plans in place to handle kids who are overweight (≥85–94th percentile BMI) and obese (≥95th percentile BMI); for instance, to track blood glucose levels over time if there's a family history of diabetes or flag charts of overweight children to remind the doctor of their heightened risk for obesity

- Onsite teams of nurses, physicians, and administrative staff dedicated to childhood obesity prevention and treatment.[1]

117. What should I expect my doctor to do?

Your doctor can serve as an ally and guide in the fight against obesity. Some of his or her key responsibilities are to:

- Assess all children 2–18 years of age at all well-care visits
- Make a weight category diagnosis using BMI percentile
- Measure blood pressure
- Take an in-depth family history
- Assess behavior and attitudes
- Perform a thorough physical exam
- Order appropriate laboratory tests
- Monitor BMI, nutritional intake, physical activity levels, and other indicators of weight in children and adolescents
- Promote a healthy lifestyle
- Treat overweight and obesity, or arrange for treatment elsewhere (such as in specialized or community-based programs)

To learn more about your doctor's role in preventing and treating childhood obesity, visit:

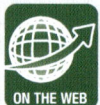

ON THE WEB

http://www.nichq.org/
documents/coan-papers-and-publications/
COANImplementationGuide62607FINAL
.pdf

118. What type of questions should my doctor ask during a medical history?

The medical history for an overweight or obese child should focus on any underlying causes, such as hypothyroidism, and whether there are any obesity-related diseases (for example, high blood pressure). The discussion should include questions about snoring or other signs of sleep problems; symptoms of diabetes, such as unusual thirst or more frequent urination; and for girls going through puberty, questions about acne, excess hairiness (hirsutism), and the onset and frequency of menstruation. The doctor should ask if your child is taking antipsychotics associated with weight gain, such as clozapine, respiridone, olanzapine, and quetiapine.

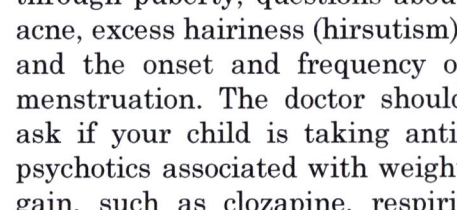

Hypothyroidism is a syndrome that results from abnormally low secretion of thyroid hormones from the thyroid gland, leading to a decrease in basal (resting) metabolic rate.

DEFINITION

The medical history should also assess risk factors for childhood obesity, such as a child's size for gestational age (large or small), parental obesity (especially maternal), maternal weight gain during pregnancy, duration of breastfeeding, and weight of siblings and more distant relatives.

119. What other information will my doctor want?

Your doctor will also want to know what your child eats. Among other information (such as whether he or she has breakfast), your clinician will want an estimate of the type and quantity of beverages consumed, how often your child eats out and where, and the type and number of snacks he or she has each day.

An activity history will include how long, how often, and how intensely your child exercises during and after school; if he or she plays team sports, bikes to and from school, walks the dog, or takes part in any other activities that burn energy. Your doctor will also want an estimate of how much time each day is spent sitting around watching television, texting, or playing computer games.

You'll also hear questions about your neighborhood, such as whether it's safe to go out and play, if there are parks nearby with playground equipment, or if your child has access to a recreation center, pool, or gym.

120. Why does my child's doctor need all this information?

Your child's doctor wants this information for several reasons. One is to rule out underlying conditions or reasons for overweight or obesity. Another is to identify diet or physical activity factors that contribute to weight gain. A third is to find out if you or your family can modify some or all of those behaviors.

Medical history is relevant information about a patient's past, present, and future health. The medical history is an account of all medical events and problems a person has experienced and is an important tool in their care.

To suggest realistic changes, a physician needs to know about the resources patients and their families have and the barriers that might stop them from following through on a plan to fight obesity. Many factors influence a child's weight, from cultural values to the distance to the nearest supermarket. The more a doctor knows, the better able he or she will be to develop a plan that will meet the specific needs of each patient and family.

121. My child is having problems sleeping. What type of screening and diagnostic tests should my doctor do?

Sleep problems are among the most serious obesity-related ailments (see Chapter 2). One common cause is obstructive sleep apnea, a condition in which breathing is interrupted throughout the night, resulting in daytime sleepiness. Symptoms include loud or unusual snoring with pauses and gasps. Another problem is obesity hypoventilation syndrome (OHS), a disorder in which poor breathing results in too much carbon dioxide (hypoventilation) and too little oxygen in the blood (hypoxemia). Many children with OHS also have obstructive sleep apnea. Both conditions are diagnosed with polysomnography, a sleep study that records certain body functions as the patient sleeps, or tries to do so.

To find out more about polysomnography, visit:

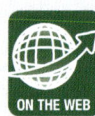 ON THE WEB

http://www.nlm.nih.gov/medlineplus/ency/article/003932.htm

To find out more about hemoglobin, visit:

ON THE WEB

http://www.nlm.nih.gov/medlineplus/ency/article/003645.htm

To learn about hematocrit, visit:

http://www.nlm.nih.gov/medlineplus/ency/article/003646.htm

To find out what CPAP is and how it works, visit:

http://www.nlm.nih.gov/medlineplus/ency/article/003646.htm

In cases of obstructive sleep apnea, enlarged tonsils and adenoids are first removed. If this approach doesn't resolve the problem, a lung doctor or pulmonologist should evaluate whether your child needs continuous positive airway pressure (CPAP) therapy during sleep. CPAP requires equipment that delivers mild air pressure to keep your child's airway open during the night.

In children with OHS, polysomnography shows elevated carbon dioxide levels. Hemoglobin, a protein in red blood cells that carries oxygen, is also tested along with hematocrit, the proportion of red blood cells in total blood volume. People with low hemoglobin feel fatigued; those with a low hematocrit are anemic. Those who have OHS will need CPAP until substantial weight loss relieves the condition.[2]

122. How should obese children be screened for gastrointestinal problems and how often?

Common gastrointestinal problems in obese children include nonalcoholic fatty liver disease (NAFLD), gallstones, and cholecystitis (inflammation of the gallbladder). Elevated blood levels of serum alanine aminotransferase (ALT), a liver enzyme, are used to screen for NAFLD. Ultrasound and other imaging methods can identify gallstones and inflammation of the gallbladder.

They can also show changes that indicate advanced NAFLD, such as nonalcoholic steatohepatitis (NASH), which is fat in the liver along with inflammation and damage. A liver biopsy can determine degrees of inflammation or fibrosis (scarring of the liver).

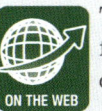

To find out more about fatty liver disease and childhood obesity, watch:

https://www.youtube.com/watch?v=VEtTcO4guzE

ALT should be screened biannually starting at 10 years of age for children with a BMI at or above the 95th percentile. Children with a BMI in the 85th to 94th percentile who have other risk factors should also be screened every two years. Results that are twice the normal level (> 60 units per liter of blood) on two occasions should prompt consultation with a pediatric liver specialist.[2]

Alanine aminotransferase (ALT) is an enzyme normally found in liver cells. It's released into the bloodstream when the liver is damaged (for example, by NAFLD), and can be identified with a blood test.

123. Diabetes runs in my family. How often should my child be tested?

Severely obese children and adolescents often have hyperinsulinemia or glucose intolerance. Hyperinsulinemia is also known as pre-diabetes or insulin resistance. It's a condition in which the body fails to use insulin to remove glucose from the blood, resulting in higher levels of insulin than normal. Glucose intolerance is higher than normal blood glucose levels or hyperglycemia.

Hyperinsulinemia is a high level of insulin in the plasma due to increased secretion of insulin by the pancreas.
Hyperglycemia is an abnormally high blood glucose level beyond the normal range (roughly 70–150 mg/100 ml of blood).

Early screening for diabetes can detect these conditions and identify diabetes before symptoms appear. Appropriate interventions during this period can prevent or delay onset of the disease and its complications. Children and adolescents who are overweight (BMI ≥ 85th percentile for age and gender) and have any two other risk factors (for example, hypertension plus a first-degree relative with diabetes) should be screened every three years. Children and adolescents who are obese (BMI ≥ 95th percentile for age and gender) should be screened without regard to risk factors. Testing should start at puberty or at 10 years of age.[3] A fasting glucose level ≥ 126 mg/dL or a casual (without regard to time of last meal) glucose level of ≥ 200 mg/dL indicate diabetes and require a referral to a pediatric endocrinologist.

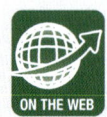

To find out more about more about the relationship between obesity and type 2 diabetes, visit:

http://theweightofthenation.hbo
.com/watch/bonus-shorts/
obesity-and-type-2-diabetes

124. My father had heart disease. Should my child be screened for this?

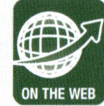

To find out more about childhood obesity and high blood pressure, visit:

http://www.heart.org/HEARTORG/
Conditions/HighBlood
Pressure/UnderstandYourRiskfor
HighBloodPressure/High-Blood-Pressure-
in-Children_UCM_301868_Article.jsp

Cholesterol and triglycerides are important fats in the blood. Cholesterol is an essential component of cell membranes, brain and nerve cells, and bile. It helps the body absorb fats and fat-soluble vitamins. The body uses cholesterol to make vitamin D and hormones such as estrogen, testosterone, and cortisol. The body can produce all the cholesterol that it needs, but it also gets it from food. Triglycerides are contained in fat cells. They can be broken down and used to provide energy for the body's metabolic processes, including growth.

Your doctor should check your child's blood pressure at every visit. His or her office should be equipped with large cuffs, including thigh cuffs that allow for accurate assessment of blood pressure in severely obese children and adolescents.

Lipids are fats in the blood, and lipid abnormalities are common in obese children and adolescents. To make sure your child isn't at risk for heart disease, your doctor should take a fasting lipid profile for children whose BMI is ≥85th percentile, even if there are no other risk factors. Total cholesterol levels of < 170 mg/dL are in the normal range. Levels of 170–199 mg/dL are in the borderline category, and high cholesterol is defined as lipid levels ≥ 200 mg/dL.

Low-density lipoprotein cholesterol is the "bad" cholesterol. Levels of < 110 mg/dL are acceptable. Levels of 110–129 mg/dL are borderline, and a level ≥ 130 mg/dL is high. High-density lipoprotein is the "good" cholesterol. Abnormal high-density lipoprotein (≤ 40 mg/dL) and triglyceride levels (≥ 110 mg/dL for adolescents) respond to increased physical activity.

 Lipids can be a significant risk factor for coronary artery disease. High levels can be inherited or acquired (largely through lifestyle, especially a high fat diet). Hyperlipidemia has no symptoms, and can only be diagnosed by a screening blood test. Treatment requires changes in diet or the use of lipid-lowering drugs (statins). These two approaches have led to reductions in disability and death.

Your child may need to see a pediatric cardiologist or lipid specialist if blood fat levels are very high and do not respond to changes in diet. These doctors can assess the risks and benefits of medication.

125. What screening tests should my doctor perform and what findings are considered normal?

Your doctor can rule out diabetes, lipid problems, and other comorbidities (obesity-related conditions) with screening tests. The most common are shown in the following table.

Screening tests for the more common obesity comorbidities

COMORBIDITY	CASE DETECTION TESTS (ABNORMAL VALUES)
Pre-diabetes	
1) Impaired fasting plasma glucose (verify fasting status)	Fasting plasma glucose (> 100 mg/dL)
2) Impaired glucose tolerance (if an OGTT* is used)	2-hour glucose > 140 but < 200 mg/dL
Diabetes mellitus	Fasting plasma glucose > 126 mg/dL or random value > 200 mg/dL (If an OGTT is used, 2 hour glucose > 200) If asymptomatic, repeated abnormal values on another occasion are required

Continued

Continued

COMORBIDITY	CASE DETECTION TESTS (ABNORMAL VALUES)
Dyslipidemia	Fasting (12–14 hours) lipids
	Triglycerides > 110 mg/dL (75th percentile); ≥ 160 mg/dL (90th percentile)
	LDL cholesterol ≥ 110 mg/dL (75th percentile); ≥ 130 mg/dL (90th percentile)
	Total cholesterol ≥ 180 mg/m/dL (75th percentile); ≥ 200 mg/dL (90th percentile)
	HDL cholesterol ≤ 35 mg/dL (10th percentile); < 40 mg/dL (25th percentile)
Hypertension	Blood pressure > 90th percentile (standardized according to sex, age, and height percentile)
NAFLD	Alanine aminotransferase (ALT) > two standard deviations above the average for the laboratory

*OGTT, oral glucose tolerance test

SOURCE: The Endocrine Society's Clinical Guidelines. Prevention and Treatment of Pediatric Obesity: An Endocrine Society Clinical Practice Guideline Based on Expert Opinion, https://www.endocrine.org/~/media/endosociety/Files/Publications/Clinical%20Practice%20Guidelines/FINAL-Standalone-Pediatric-Obesity-Guideline.pdf

126. My child cries when she looks in the mirror. What can my doctor do to help?

Stigma, bullying, isolation, and other social problems associated with obesity can take a high toll on your child's self-esteem and quality of life. Depression can precede or result from obesity. Clinicians should look for flat affect (lack of emotion), anxiety, body dissatisfaction, excess eating, fatigue, and difficulty sleeping. Children and adolescents with binge eating or purging behavior should be evaluated for eating disorders.

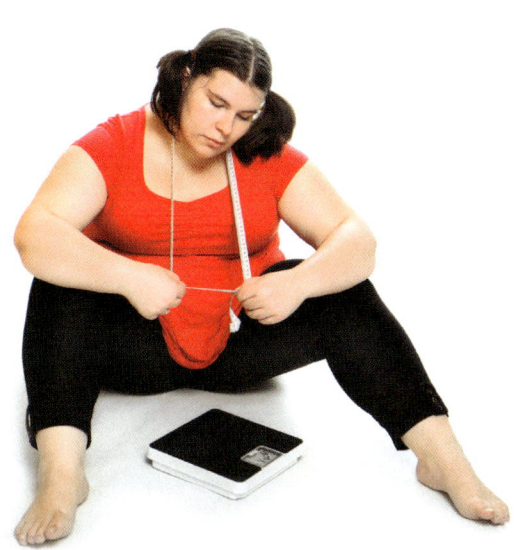

◀ **FIGURE 9.1**
Obesity can cause
isolation and
despair. © Kletr

SOURCE: Shutterstock

Treatment Options for Childhood Obesity

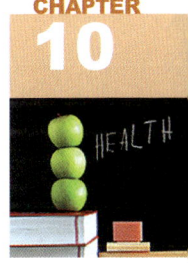

CHAPTER
10

Treatment of severe obesity in children is challenging. Moderate weight loss of 5–10% of initial body weight can improve or reverse most obesity-related illnesses, yet even modest goals can be hard to achieve and even more difficult to sustain.

127. My teenager really tries hard to lose weight but keeps regaining it. Why is this happening?

Weight loss efforts can be subverted by the body's own responses. Weight loss increases ghrelin, the hunger hormone. Leptin and other hormones that tell the brain that the stomach's full decrease. Resting metabolic rate (the energy your body uses to perform vital

NOTE

Eating less and being more active are the only ways to keep excess weight off. To indefinitely maintain weight loss, an adolescent must continue to restrict energy intake or increase energy output.

To learn more about ghrelin, visit:

http://www.yourhormones.info/hormones/ghrelin.aspx

To find out more about leptin, visit:

http://www.yourhormones.info/hormones/leptin.aspx

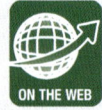

Resting metabolic rate is the energy required to perform vital body functions, such as respiration and heart rate, while the body is at rest. About 50–75% of daily energy expenditure can be attributed to resting metabolic rate.

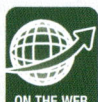

To find out more about why children are unlikely to outgrow excess weight, visit:

http://consumer.healthday.com/kids-health-information-23/misc-kid-s-health-news-435/kids-unlikely-to-outgrow-baby-fat-684338.html

The main goal of obesity treatment is to improve long-term physical health through permanent changes in lifestyle habits.

To find out more about the emotional toll of obesity, visit:

http://www.healthychildren.org/English/health-issues/conditions/obesity/Pages/The-Emotional-Toll-of-Obesity.aspx

body functions) falls as the pounds drop off, causing the body to burn fewer calories than normal. Many other cues, such as reward and emotional factors, also play a role in how much food is consumed. Eating less and being more active are the only ways to keep excess weight off. To indefinitely maintain weight loss, an adolescent must continue to restrict energy intake or increase energy output.

128. My child is overweight. Can't he outgrow the excess fat?

It depends on whether he can maintain his current weight as he grows. To do that, calories in have to equal calories burned; your child needs to balance eating and exercise until his height catches up to his weight. This is no easy task. Overweight 5-year-old children face four times the risk of being obese at age 14 compared to their normal-weight peers, and severely obese children have a high likelihood of becoming severely obese adults.

129. Is weight loss the only goal of obesity treatment?

The main goal of obesity treatment is to improve long-term physical health through permanent changes in lifestyle habits. For some children, new behaviors alone will lead to improved weight (either weight loss or maintenance during growth). Others might need a behavior modification program or some other kind of help to turn new activities into a routine part of daily life. Emotional well-being is also a very important objective of treatment.

130. What's the best kind of intervention to treat childhood obesity?

No single approach is the best way to treat childhood obesity; the nature, format, intensity, frequency, and length of any program depend on the needs, cultural influences, and circumstances of the child and his or her family. Some youngsters will respond best to individual case management, where they have private, age-appropriate conversations with clinicians and dietitians on such subjects as goal setting, diet, exercise, and readiness.

Others will do well in community- or school-based group interventions. These can include physical activity sessions, educational grocery store visits, parent-only meetings, family cooking courses, and group counseling.[1] Depending on their BMI, certain children might need counseling plus medication. Weight loss surgery might be the best option for those with severe obesity.

 No single approach is the best way to treat childhood obesity; the nature, format, intensity, frequency, and length of any program depend on the needs, cultural influences, and circumstances of the child and his or her family.

131. What are the treatment options for children who are overweight or obese?

Intensive lifestyle modification is the first step to all treatments for overweight or obese children and adolescents.

 Intensive lifestyle modification is the first step to all treatments for overweight or obese children and adolescents.

Effective comprehensive weight management programs include counseling and other components that target diet and physical activity. They offer a wide range of behavior change strategies, such as self-monitoring, stimulus control techniques (for example, not bringing ice cream into the house), positive reinforcement, problem-solving skills, social support, and relapse prevention.

Programs for younger children involve parents. Their participation and modeling of healthy behaviors are crucial

Parental involvement is essential for success. Their participation and modeling of healthy behaviors are crucial components of pediatric weight management.

components of pediatric weight management. Youth in weight loss programs that include parents have improved body composition and metabolic factors, such as lipids.

Moderate-to high-intensity programs involve more than 25 hours of contact with the child and/or the family over a 6-month period. These interventions can help youngsters achieve a lower BMI and maintain it for at least a year after the start of the program. Low-intensity interventions, defined as 25 contact hours or fewer over a 6-month period, do not lead to significant weight loss.[4]

Even with success, weight regain can occur after the active phase of an intervention ends. Lack of continued exercise may be a major factor. The odds for weight regain are twofold greater in patients who return to a sedentary lifestyle.[5] Other reasons include biological changes in hunger and satiety hormones or pressures at home. In families with economic problems, weight control may not be a top priority compared with other issues they face.

Intensive lifestyle interventions with long-term maintenance, such as individual or group counseling, physical fitness classes, or some other type of ongoing contact are more likely to produce weight loss. In addition, the national drive to fight childhood obesity has led to more treatment options through school-, faith-, and community-based programs that teach children about healthy living, physical activity, and weight loss.

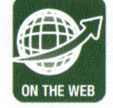

To learn more about lifestyle interventions for the treatment of overweight and obesity, visit:

http://www.cdc.gov/obesity/childhood/researchproject.html

In general, lifestyle interventions that include a dietary component plus exercise and/or behavioral therapy can be an effective treatment for childhood obesity. Compared to standard care or self-help, such programs can lead to significant and clinically meaningful reductions in weight and improvements in other measures of health.

132. Can you give me some examples of weight loss programs for children and adolescents?

Weight loss programs are individually designed to promote weight management and healthy living in children and adolescents.

No two are exactly the same. They take place in various settings including schools, childcare facilities, YMCA sites, church groups, and neighborhoods. Environmental-level interventions focus on enforcement of policies or legislation as well as changes to the environment (such as creating parks, playgrounds, basketball and tennis courts, and swimming pools). Some examples of interventions include:

- The Traffic Light Diet, a calorie-controlled approach in which foods are color-coded according to their calorie density per average serving: green for low-calorie foods that can be eaten freely, yellow for moderate-calorie foods that can be eaten occasionally, and red for high-calorie foods that should be eaten very infrequently
- A short-term, six-month community-based program in which children and parents attended eighteen two-hour group education and exercise sessions twice weekly in sports centers and schools, followed by a twelve-week free family swimming pass
- A peer-mentoring approach in which older elementary school students (9–12 years old) teach younger ones (6–8 years of age) using lesson plans that focus on physical activity, healthy eating, self-esteem, and body image
- A two-month community-based intensive exercise training program (four times per week, ninety minutes per session) combined with dietary restrictions (500 calories per day less than reported baseline energy intake)
- A comprehensive program that teaches children what healthy food is and where it comes from, provides hands-on opportunities to grow fresh food in school gardens, and works with farmers, chefs, and school food service personnel to get nutritious foods onto lunch menus.

133. How can I find a lifestyle intervention for my child?

Good places to look include those where interventions are planned, funded, or carried out (schools, YMCAs, local churches, hospitals, state and local departments of public health, and the offices of community leaders, such as mayors and local officials). Your pediatrician can help you locate

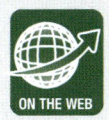

ON THE WEB

To find out more about what programs might be available in your area, visit:

https://foodcorps.org/

http://www.sparkpe.org/about-us/

a program. You might also call the Centers for Disease Control and Prevention at 800-CDC-INFO (800-232-4636).

134. Are there any drugs my child can take to help him lose weight?

Unless it's used as part of a structured lifestyle modification program, pharmacotherapy (the use of medications) alone is not an effective treatment for obesity. It can lead to modest short-term improvement in the weight of children aged twelve and older, but weight regain is common, especially after a child stops taking the drug. Despite these limitations, the use of medications to treat pediatric obesity is becoming more common. The number of options is limited, however, and their safety and efficacy are uncertain.

To date, drugs tested for treatment of childhood obesity include sibutramine, orlistat, metformin, and exenatide. The most effective of these, sibutramine, was removed from the U.S. market due to cardiovascular concerns. Metformin and exenatide are used off-label (without the approval of the U.S. Food and Drug Administration [FDA]). Orlistat is the only medication that's been approved by the FDA for weight loss in those aged twelve or older.

135. What is orlistat and how does it work?

Orlistat is a lipase inhibitor; it blocks the absorption of fats, which then pass through the intestine and are excreted in the feces. It's administered three times per day and produces modest weight loss in obese adolescents. Although it has a good safety profile, its side effects have prevented widespread use. Common problems include oily spotting on underwear, urgent bowel movements, and stomach pain. Those who take orlistat also need a supplement to replace water-soluble vitamins that get excreted along with fats.

To find out more about orlistat, visit:

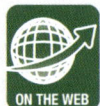
ON THE WEB

http://www.nlm.nih.gov/medlineplus/druginfo/meds/a601244.html

136. What is metformin and how does it work?

Metformin is mainly used to control blood sugar in adults with type 2 diabetes, but it has also been evaluated for its effect on weight loss in a number of studies in children and adolescents. Most of these have shown modest reductions in body weight and/or BMI. Metformin is taken by mouth and is available in two forms: a shorter-acting tablet taken twice per day and an extended-release version taken once a day. The drug has a good safety record. Common side effects (mostly nausea and vomiting) are usually mild.

In adults, metformin not only helps with weight loss, it also delays the onset of type 2 diabetes. Teens with severe obesity who are at risk of type 2 diabetes—those with an elevated HbA1c (a blood test that measures the average level of blood sugar over the previous three months) or a family history of type 2 diabetes—might benefit from this medication. However, studies have yet to be performed in adolescents with severe obesity (BMI $\geq$ 120% of the 95th percentile or $\geq$ 35 kg/m^2).

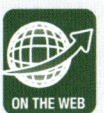

To learn more about metformin, visit:

http://www.nlm.nih.gov/medlineplus/druginfo/meds/a696005.html

137. What is exenatide and how does it work?

Exenatide increases feeling of fullness and suppresses appetite. In children and adolescents with severe obesity, it produces modest reductions in BMI and improves fasting insulin resistance. The longer it's taken the more weight is lost. The drug is delivered via injection. Side effects include mild to moderate nausea and vomiting. More studies are needed to evaluate the safety and efficacy of exenatide treatment in obese children and teens.[6]

Insulin resistance is the diminished effectiveness of insulin in lowering blood sugar levels.

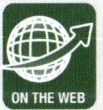

To find out more about exenatide, visit:

http://www.nlm.nih.gov/medlineplus/druginfo/meds/a605034.html

138. What's the bottom line on weight loss drugs?

In general, the use of weight loss drugs in obese children and adolescents has been disappointing. Reductions in weight or BMI have been modest with relatively little impact on cardiometabolic risk factors, such as hypertension and cholesterol levels. If used, medications should be tailored to the individual patient, with family history a major consideration.

The main objective of drug therapy is to prevent obesity-related illnesses in patients with a BMI ≥ 95th percentile. In general, medications should not be given to children with a BMI below that level. In overweight youth (BMI > 85th but < 95th percentile), it should be limited to those with severe comorbidities who have not responded to lifestyle interventions. In all cases, the benefits of taking a drug should exceed the risks.

The main objective of drug therapy is to prevent obesity-related illnesses in patients with a BMI ≥95th percentile.

NOTE

139. My child is extremely obese. Would she be a candidate for weight loss surgery?

Over the past decade, weight loss surgery has become more broadly accepted for a select group of severely obese adolescents. To be considered for bariatric surgery, a teen has to have reached physical and psychological maturity, and have a BMI that is either ≥ 120% of the 95th percentile or ≥ 35 kg/m² (whichever is lower). They also need to show an inability to lose weight after six months of supervised participation in two separate behavioral or medical weight loss programs.

Weight loss or bariatric surgery should only be considered if there is a psychological evaluation that confirms the stability and competence of the family unit. The patient also has to demonstrate that he or she is emotionally stable, well-informed, and has the motivation and ability to adhere to strict postoperative diet and physical activity requirements.[5]

140. Who should perform weight loss surgery?

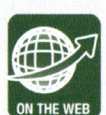

To find out more about weight loss surgery, visit:

http://childrensnational.org/departments/bariatric-surgery-program

ON THE WEB

The operation should be performed by an experienced weight loss surgeon in a medical facility with a multidisciplinary weight loss team that can provide a preoperative evaluation and long-term care of the patient and family. Adolescents who undergo weight loss surgery require lifelong medical and nutritional follow-up, especially to ensure that they get adequate vitamins and minerals. They also need extensive and ongoing counseling. Without such support, patients tend to regain their weight over time.

141. What kinds of weight loss surgeries are performed on adolescents?

Weight loss surgery is the most effective treatment for obesity. Compared with intensive lifestyle intervention, with or without medication, the superiority of surgery is now well accepted.

There are two basic types of bariatric surgeries: restrictive and malabsorptive/restrictive. Restrictive surgery shrinks the size of the stomach. Restrictive/malabsorptive operations change the size of the stomach as well as the way food is digested by physically removing or bypassing part of the digestive tract. This makes it harder for the body to absorb calories.

Four procedures are performed on adolescents: laparoscopic adjustable gastric banding, Roux-en-Y gastric bypass, vertical sleeve gastrectomy, and biliopancreatic diversion, with or without duodenal switch.

142. How does gastric banding work?

Gastric banding is the least invasive surgery. It uses an inflatable band to divide the stomach into two parts: a smaller upper pouch and a larger lower one. The two sections remain connected, but the channel between them is much smaller. This slows down the emptying of the upper pouch and physically restricts the amount of food your child can take in at any given meal.

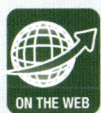

To find out more about adjustable gastric banding, visit:

http://www.hopkins-medicine.org/healthlibrary/test_procedures/gastroenterology/laparoscopic_adjustable_gastric_banding_135,63/

143. What is Roux-en-Y gastric bypass?

Laparoscopic Roux-en-Y gastric bypass combines restrictive and malabsorptive approaches. The operation divides the stomach into two parts, sealing off the upper section from the lower one. The surgeon connects the upper stomach directly to the lower part of the small intestine. Food then passes out of the body quickly, reducing the amount of calories that can be absorbed.

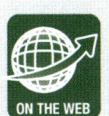

To learn more about Roux-en-Y gastric bypass, visit:

http://www.webmd.com/diet/weight-loss-surgery/gastric-bypass

144. What does the surgeon do in a sleeve gastrectomy?

Laparoscopic sleeve gastrectomy is another form of restrictive surgery. The operation removes about 75% of the stomach. What remains is a narrow tube or sleeve that connects to the intestines. Sometimes, laparoscopic sleeve gastrectomy is the first step in a sequence of operations for severely obese individuals. It can be followed by gastric bypass or biliopancreatic diversion (see below) if more weight loss is needed. In most cases, though, it's the only surgery needed.

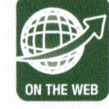

To learn more about laparoscopic sleeve gastrectomy, visit:

http://www.obesityaction.org/wp-content/uploads/Gastric-Sleeve.pdf

ON THE WEB

145. I've never heard of biliopancreatic diversion. What is that?

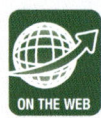

To find out more about biliopancreatic diversion with duodenal switch, watch:

ON THE WEB

http://www.mayoclinic.org/tests-procedures/bariatric-surgery/multimedia/biliopancreatic-diversion/vid-20084649

Biliopancreatic diversion is a more drastic version of gastric bypass, and is only used as a last resort. As much as 70% of the stomach is removed, and even more of the small intestine is bypassed.

A less extreme version of this procedure is biliopancreatic diversion with duodenal switch. This operation is more involved than gastric bypass, but it removes less of the stomach and bypasses less of the small intestine.

146. What happens if a severely obese child doesn't like the idea of weight loss surgery?

About 4.7% of U.S. children 6–11 years of age and 6.3% of adolescents aged 12–17 years have severe obesity.[7] They will almost always remain in the obese range, and 65% of them will have class III obesity (BMI $\geq$ 40 kg/m^2) as adults. They'll have a significantly greater risk of cardiovascular disease compared with children who are less obese, and have more health complications and higher mortality compared with those who become obese as adults.[7]

Approximately 4.7% of U.S. children 6–11 years of age and 6.3% of adolescents aged 12–17 years have severe obesity; 65% of them will have class III obesity (BMI $\geq$ 40 kg/m^2) as adults.

NOTE

147. What can bariatric surgery do that a good intervention can't?

Only a small proportion of adolescents with class III obesity will receive surgery, but those who do gain many benefits. Unlike dieting, which triggers responses such as hunger and cravings, certain weight loss surgeries reboot the set point weight to a "normal" level. Adolescents are more content with less food, and they achieve major, long-term weight loss. Like any surgery, however, each procedure has risks and benefits.

148. What are the risks and benefits of laparoscopic adjustable gastric banding?

On the up side, laparoscopic gastric banding is simpler to do and safer than gastric bypass and other operations. Recovery from laparoscopic banding is faster than from other surgeries, and the procedure is reversible. The band is connected to an opening just beneath the skin in the stomach, and can easily be loosened or tightened by either injecting or removing saline solution with a needle.

However, gastric banding is being used far less frequently. Although the most common side effect is vomiting, which results from eating too much food too quickly, weight loss produced by this procedure is less dramatic than that seen with alternative surgeries. Patients are also more likely to regain weight over time.

Complications are also common, especially on a long-term basis. The band can slip, become too loose, or leak. Infection is a risk, and sometimes further surgeries are needed. Nonetheless, life-threatening complications are unlikely.

149. What are the risks and benefits of laparoscopic gastric bypass?

Laparoscopic Roux-en-Y gastric bypass produces swift and dramatic weight loss, mostly in the first six months after surgery. The reduction lasts for many years, and the procedure restores normal cardiometabolic markers of health, such as blood pressure and lipids. Type 2 diabetes improves or goes away within hours after surgery. Other obesity-related comorbidities, such as high cholesterol, arthritis, and sleep apnea get better as well. Roux-en-Y gastric bypass also improves quality of life.

However, the procedure is not without risks. Gastric bypass impairs the body's ability to absorb food. This causes the rapid weight loss, but it can also put a patient at risk of nutritional deficiencies. The loss of calcium can lead to osteoporosis, and iron losses can lead to anemia. Adolescents need to be very careful about what they eat, and take supplements for the rest of their lives. The procedure is also irreversible.

Dumping syndrome, a complication usually triggered by sugary or high-carbohydrate foods, is another problem. Food is "dumped" from the stomach into the intestines before proper digestion. About 85% of patients suffer symptoms that include nausea, bloating, pain, sweating, weakness, and diarrhea.

To learn more about the risks and complications associated with laparoscopic gastric banding and gastric bypass surgery, visit:

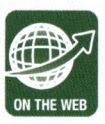

https://weightloss.clevelandclinic.org/images/file/Risks%20and%20complications%20of%20bariatric%20surgery.pdf

Gastric bypass is a more complex procedure than gastric banding. Complications include possible leaks, hernias, and gallstones. The 30-day mortality rate is 0.14%.

150. What are the risks and benefits of sleeve gastrectomy?

Sleeve gastrectomy is now the most widely recommended surgery for weight loss. It delivers all the benefits of Roux-en-Y gastric bypass without nutritional deficits or dumping. It's also less risky to perform. In people with high BMIs, sleeve gastrectomies result in an average weight loss of greater than 50% of excess weight. If the procedure doesn't deliver expected results, a limb that provides nourishment (an alimentary limb) can be added to bypass more of the duodenum. This results in greater weight loss. It also elicits hormones needed to prevent type 2 diabetes and improves or resolves other obesity-related conditions.

To learn more about the risks and complications of sleeve gastrectomy, visit:

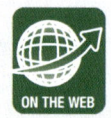

http://asmbs.org/resources/studies-weigh-in-on-safety-and-effectiveness-of-newer-bariatric-and-metabolic-surgery-procedure

Like gastric bypass, sleeve gastrectomies are irreversible and carry the normal risks of surgery (infection and blood clots). Sleeve leaks are also a concern.

151. Is biliopancreatic diversion a risky procedure?

Biliopancreatic diversion can take off more weight faster than gastric bypass: 70–80% of excess weight in the long-term. However, the procedure is more involved than Roux-en-Y gastric bypass and the risk of nutritional deficiencies is more serious. It also causes dumping syndrome, but the duodenal switch can reduce that risk. Biliopancreatic diversion is one of the most complicated and high-risk bariatric surgeries.

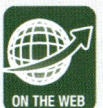

http://www.bariatricsin-seattle.com/procedures/combined-surgeries/biliopancreatic-diversion-duodenal-switch/

152. Are we getting anywhere in our fight against childhood obesity?

Childhood obesity seems to have stabilized, but the crisis is far from over. One in three American children and teens remains overweight or obese. Parents are the key to progress. However, they routinely underestimate their offprings's weight, or are not concerned about it despite the very high toll obesity exacts on the health and well-being of those who suffer from it.

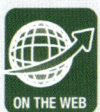

To find out how America's doing in the fight against obesity, see Video 10.1 Childhood Obesity-Are We Winning?

Preventing childhood obesity is easier than treating it. A healthy pregnancy can lay the foundation for future fitness. From there, parents can protect their children from our obesogenic environment by engaging as a family in healthy eating and physical activity.

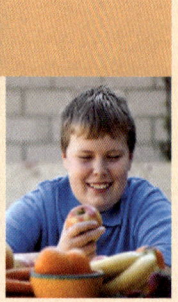

References and Endnotes

CHAPTER 9

1.   Vine M., Hargreaves M.B., Briefel R.R., Orfield C. (2013). *Expanding the Role of Primary Care in the Prevention and Treatment of Childhood Obesity: A Review of Clinic- and Community-Based Recommendations and Interventions.* J Obes, 2013:172035.

2.   Barlow S.E., Expert Committee. (2007). *Expert Committee Recommendations Regarding the Prevention, Assessment, and Treatment of Child and Adolescent Overweight and Obesity: Summary Report.* Pediatrics, 120 Suppl 4:S164-192.

3.   U.S. Department of Health and Human Services, Agency for Healthcare Quality and Research. (2011). *Clinical Practice Guideline: Screening Children and Adolescents for Type 2 Diabetes Mellitus in Primary Care.* Available at: http://www .guideline.gov/content.aspx?id=34047. Accessed July 26, 2014.

CHAPTER 10

1.   Vine M., Hargreaves M.B., Briefel R.R., Orfield C. (2013). *Expanding the Role of Primary Care in the Prevention and Treatment of Childhood Obesity: A Review of Clinic- and Community-Based Recommendations and Interventions.* J Obes, 2013:172035.

2.   Barlow S.E., Expert Committee. (2007). *Expert Committee Recommendations Regarding the Prevention, Assessment, and Treatment of Child and Adolescent Overweight and Obesity: Summary Report.* Pediatrics, 120 Suppl 4:S164-192.

3.   U.S. Department of Health and Human Services, Agency for Healthcare Quality and Research. (2011). *Clinical Practice Guideline: Screening Children and Adolescents for Type 2 Diabetes Mellitus in Primary Care.* Available at: http://www .guideline.gov/content.aspx?id=34047. Accessed July 26, 2014.

4.   U.S. Preventive Services Task Force, Barton M. (2010). *Screening for obesity in children and adolescents: U.S. Preventive Services Task Force Recommendation Statement.* Pediatrics, 125:361-367.

5.   August G.P., Caprio S., Fennoy I., et al. (2008). *Prevention and Treatment of Pediatric Obesity: An Endocrine Society Clinical Practice Guideline Based on Expert Opinion.* J Clin Endocrinol Metab, 93:4576-4599.

6. Kelly A.S., Barlow S.E., Rao G., et al. (2013). Severe Obesity in Children and Adolescents: Identification, Associated Health Risks, and Treatment Approaches: A Scientific Statement From the American Heart Association. Circulation, 128:1689-1712.

7. Xanthakos S., Inge T.H.. (2014). UpToDate.*Surgical Management of Severe Obesity in Adolescents*. Available at: http://www.uptodate.com/contents/surgical-management-of-severe-obesity-in-adolescents#H7607783. Accessed August 3, 2014.

On the Web

Visit the following Web sites for more information on Childhood Obesity.

Chapter 1. Childhood Obesity and Its Causes

Video 1.1
Be smart. Be well. What Is It? [Internet]; 2014 [cited February 10, 2014]. Podcast: 3:02. Available from: http://www.besmartbewell .com/childhood-obesity/what-is-it.htm

Video 1.2
Hofmeester F. The Mommy Files. *Video: Watch a girl grow up in in 2 minutes* 2012. Available at: http://blog.sfgate .com/sfmoms/2012/04/23/video-watch-a-girl-grow-up-in-two-minutes/

Chapter 2. Childhood Obesity and Health

Video 2.1
Childhood Obesity
http://www.pennmedicine.org/encyclopedia/em_DisplayAnima-tion.aspx?gcid=000038&ptid=57

Video 2.2
Finding Balance
http://www.cdc.gov/CDCTV/FindingBalance/

Chapter 3. Assessing Risk for Childhood Obesity

Video 3.1 – BMI Rebound: An Obesity Clue
http://www.healthychildren.org/English/health-issues/conditions/obesity/pages/BMI-Rebound-An-Obesity-Clue .aspx

Chapter 4. Preventing Obesity in Infants (0 to 12 Months)

Video 4.1 10 tips for breastfeeding success
http://www.babycenter.com/2_10-tips-for-breastfeeding-success_10326780.bc

Chapter 6. Preventing Obesity in Preschool Children

Video 6.1 Making Health Easier: Healthy Habits in Childcare.
http://www.cdc.gov/CDCTV/ChildObese/index.html

Chapter 7. Preventing Obesity in Middle Childhood

Video 7.1
Children and Adolescents: The Physical Activity Guidelines in Action
http://www.cdc.gov/healthyyouth/multimedia/videos
.htm#1

Chapter 8. Preventing Obesity in Adolescence

Video 8.1 Parents are the Key to Safe Teen Drivers
http://www.cdc.gov/CDCTV/SafeTeenDrivers/index.html
Video 8.2 Finding Balance
http://www.cdc.gov/CDCTV/FindingBalance/index.html

Index

V

Vitamin D, 53, 63

W

Weight loss
   cardiometabolic risk factors,
      99, 102
   efforts, 93–94
   FDA, 98
   metformin, 99
   programs, 96–97
World Health Organization
   (WHO), 4